Advanced Surgical Knot Tying

Knots for the General, Orthopedic, and Laparoscopic Surgeon

Philo Calhoun MD, FACS

Copyright 2023. Philo Calhoun MD

Forward

It gives me great pleasure to introduce Dr. Philo Calhoun's instructional book on suturing and knot tying! Such information is in great demand for medical students and even residents interested in learning some additional useful knots! I'm looking forward to being able to give this reference to learners.

I had the pleasure of meeting Dr. Calhoun when he came to work with us and our Oregon Health Sciences and University (OHSU) residents and students rotating at the VAMC. He has a long career dedicated to helping those in need, from working with the Indian Health Service to our veterans. He himself is a veteran. He's also a renaissance man, being an accomplished pianist. I have fond memories of him bringing in chicken breasts to help people learn rhomboid flaps, and he's a natural teacher. In fact, he earned the much coveted Surgery Resident Teaching Award at OHSU, despite his only being with us a couple of years. He clearly made an impression on our learners. I'm happy to have his teaching continue through this book! Now, while he's working with his herding dogs and spending time with his wonderful wife Lisa and his children and grandchildren, this instructional reference will continue his teaching legacy! Thanks Philo!

Karen Kwong, MD, FACS

Professor of Surgery Oregon Health and Sciences University, Residency Associate Program Director, Chief of General Surgery Division Portland VA Medical Center.

Preface

This book was initially designed as a handout to enable surgical residents to tie knots more effectively. Having taught medical students, medics in the military, and family practice and surgical residents, I have often had to correct my students' knot-tying. Loose knots may result in sutures pulling out of tissue, breaking, or untying. The consequences to patients are often serious, requiring re-operations or prolonged healing. It is common for surgeons in various specialties to tie knots that they believe are secure but are weak or loose. A 2013 article from the Mayo Clinic [1] reported that almost 80% of knots tied by surgical attendings were not tied flat.

Over the past few decades, suture materials have changed, and the use of minimally invasive laparoscopic and arthroscopic surgery has expanded. Knot-tying techniques require modification for these new sutures and procedures. Suture materials have evolved over the past several decades, and knots that were secure with rougher, more reactive materials do not always reflect the best choices for the slippery sutures more commonly used today. Techniques specific to knots tied in hard-to-reach areas or those used in minimal access procedures are often different than those easily reached by one's hands.

This book was created to review both traditional and newer knots for the surgeon. It includes traditionally described tying techniques, including one-handed and two-handed Square, slip, and instrument ties. It covers the Aberdeen knot for fascial and subcuticular closures, complex nooses, semi-locking, and locking knots. It describes newer intracorporeal and extracorporeal knots useful in laparoscopic and arthroscopic surgery.

The second edition was been reformatted in a larger size with more white space for better readability. The text was extensively revised for better clarity, over 95% of the illustrations were redrawn to be photorealistic, and minor errors were corrected. Image colors were chosen to allow better discrimination when readers use greyscale devices. The text was revised to include recommendations on when to use one knot over another in specific surgical situations. The chapter on extracorporeal knot tying was substantially expanded, and several new knots useful in orthopedic surgery were added. The chapter on hand ties added instructions on tying the Surgeon's knot, Melzer, Constrictor, modified Double Constrictor, Nicky, and Outback knots.

The third edition was revised for better clarity and consistency, with a revision of all text and illustrations in the section on hand tying. Specifics of hand tying several orthopedics knots were added, as was a section on knot tying in microsurgery. References were updated with a recent literature review.

Acknowledgments

I would like to thank the surgical residents at Oregon Health & Sciences University, without whose interest, discussions, and support this book would not have been written. I was also inspired by US Navy corpsmen's dedication to learning secure knots to care for casualties on the battlefield.

I am grateful to Howard Taylor, DVM (The Vets, Salisbury, UK) for his invaluable contributions to the section on the physics of knots and the insights he had on practical applications of these principles.

I thank LaTeX-project.org for creating accessible and open-source software used in print versions of the book. For the ePub version, Oxygen XML was used with a Docbook structure. I learned many techniques for solving 3D modeling issues on the SideFx Houdini forums, which enabled me to make illustrations for this book.

Lastly, I would like to thank my wife, Annelisa Schneider, for all her help with editing multiple revisions and for putting up with incessant discussions about tying techniques and 3D graphics, and my son, Peter Calhoun, for his suggestions on expanding the section on hand ties.

viii

Contents

Chapter 1: Overview

For thousands of years, humans have fashioned rope and twine from animal hides or plant materials and used them for hunting, making clothing, and storing food [2]. Knots were developed to secure cord reliably. Hundreds of knots were invented for boating, climbing, fishing, and other activities. Before the use of sutures, the pincers of ants were sometimes used to re-approximate wounds, but sutures supplemented this practice even in ancient societies. As far back as 3000 BC, Egyptians used sutures for the burial preparation of mummies.

Archaeological evidence of needles made of bone or metal suggests that suturing of wounds dates back thousands of years. Originally, suture threads were made from plant fibers, but these were eventually replaced with strips of animal materials. The first recorded use of catgut (made from cow or sheep intestines) as a suturing material is attributed to Galen of Pergamon in the second century AD. The Indian physician Sushruta wrote about interrupted and continuous suturing techniques in 500 BC. Hippocrates, the Greek father of medicine, used the term "suture" to describe wound closure techniques in 400 BC.

In the first century AD, the Greek doctor Heraklas described sixteen knots that could be used for surgical or orthopedic procedures [3]. This included the Hercules knot, now known as the Square knot, which is fundamental to modern surgical knot tying.

Traditionally, techniques for surgical knot tying were developed for high-friction suture materials, like silk, cotton, and catgut. Recently, monofilament low-friction sutures have supplanted braided sutures for many surgical procedures. Newer knot-tying techniques have borrowed from methods used in climbing, fishing, and boating - where slippery material needs to be tied with high reliability.

Chapter 2: Suture Materials

Suture materials have varying friction coefficients and resistance to slipping and untying. Sutures can be divided into non-absorbable and absorbable, categorized by whether they are braided or monofilament, or differentiated by how much tissue reactivity or inflammation is caused by the material.

Non-absorbable sutures

Non-absorbable sutures are helpful when the body will not heal to full strength. They are used for biologic hernia surgery, vascular anastomoses, and tendon repairs. Silk has traditionally been used to ligate blood vessels, as it has excellent knot security and is easy to tie. Non-absorbable sutures can be used to close skin if they are removed before scarring occurs. An overview of suture materials is given below [4]:

Silk Silk is considered a non-absorbable material, but it degrades in tissue over two years. Silk has excellent handling and knot-tying properties. It is a braided suture.

Nylon (Ethilon - monofilament, Ethicon; Nurolon - braided, Ethicon) Nylon is available in both monofilamentous and braided forms. Nylon has high tensile strength, and although it is classified as non-absorbable, it loses tensile strength over time. Braided forms retain no tensile strength after being in tissue for six months, whereas monofilamentous forms retain two-thirds of their original strength after eleven years.

Polyester (Ethibond and Merselene, Ethicon) Polyester is a braided coated suture with high tensile strength, exemplary handling, good knot security, and low tissue reactivity. It is often blended with polyethylene (Ethibond and Mersilene).

Polypropylene (Prolene, Ethicon) Polypropylene's tensile strength is lower than that of the other synthetic non-absorbable sutures. Tissue reactivity is extremely low, and absorption does not occur if it is buried in tissue.

Absorbable sutures

Absorbable suture materials are useful to minimize infection and scarring when tissue strength during healing is not impaired. These are commonly used to close fascia or deep layers or to secure permanent mesh for hernia repairs. Ideally, an absorbable suture should maintain strength long enough to ensure sufficient strength of a wound but disappear soon afterward to minimize the suture's inflammatory properties and reduce the chance of infection (since sutures impair the host's ability to eliminate bacteria adherent to foreign materials). For skin sutures, unless excessive tension, immunosuppression, or other factors delay wound healing, strength is only required for 5-14 days. For intestinal anastomoses, the suture should maintain strength for at least two to three weeks, as intestinal leaks are most common from days 5-10. Facial sutures similarly should maintain strength for at least three weeks, as fascial dehiscence is most common within the first two weeks after surgery.

Absorbable suture strength over time is shown below [5–11]:

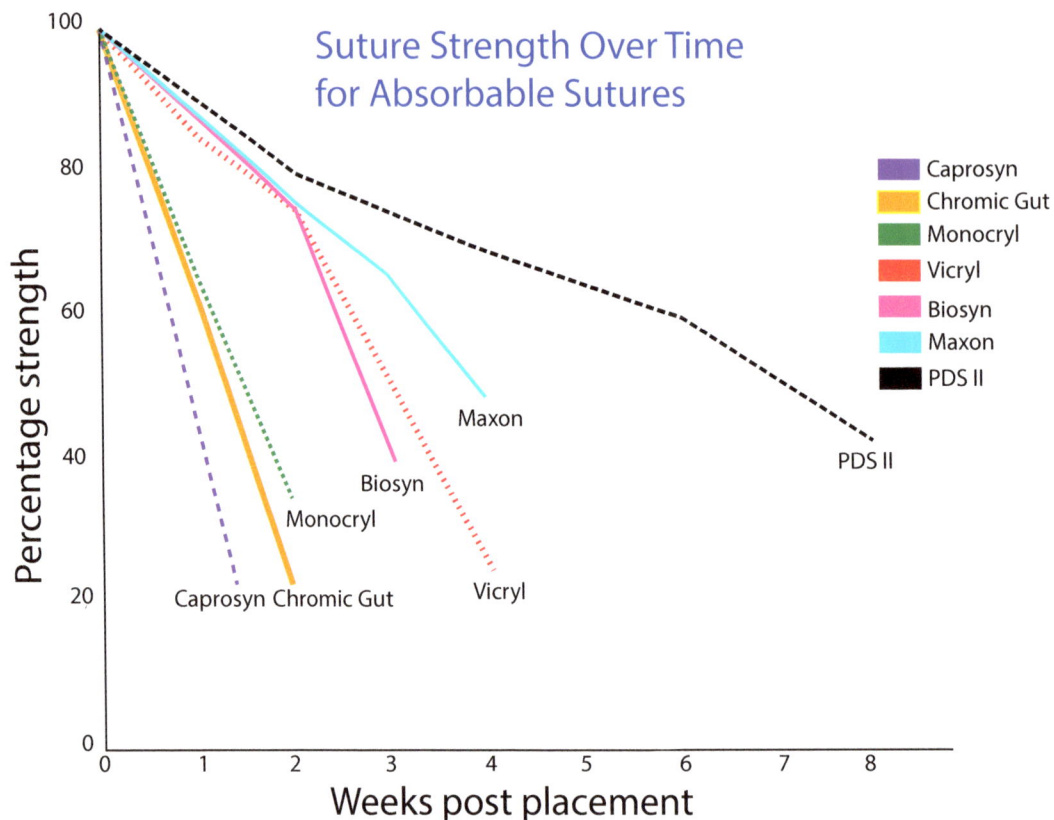

Figure 2.1: Suture strength over time

Rapidly dissolving sutures

Rapid dissolving sutures are useful for subcuticular skin closures. The rapid dissolution minimizes suture extrusion but assures apposition long enough for adequate tissue strength in healing. In either continuous or interrupted subcuticular closures, it is important to suture so that the knot is directed downwards, as even short-acting sutures take months to be absorbed completely. Of all the short-acting sutures, Biosyn has the best knot-tying properties, as the knot compresses during tying and helps prevent unraveling.

Poliglecapron (Monocryl, Ethicon) Poliglecaprone is a monofilament suture that initially has a very high tensile strength (higher than PDS II or Maxon) but after two weeks retains only 20-30% of its strength. Complete hydrolysis occurs in 90-120 days.

Glycomer 631 (Biosyn, Covidien) Glycomer 631 is a monofilament suture with greater knot security than Monocryl. It retains 75% of its tensile strength at two weeks and 40% at three weeks. Absorption is complete between 90 and 110 days.

Polyglytone 6211 (Caprosyn, Covidien) Polyglytone 6211 is a monofilament suture with rapid absorption, maintaining secure wound approximation for ten days. All tensile strength is lost by three weeks. It is completely hydrolyzed in 56 days.

Polyglactin (Vicryl, Ethicon) Polyglactin is a coated braided suture. The coating reduces drag but also reduces knot security, requiring four squared throws for knot security. It retains 60% of its tensile strength at two weeks and 8% of its original strength at four weeks. It is completely hydrolyzed after 60-90 days. Tissue reactivity is low. It is the subcutaneous suture of choice of 73% of surgical dermatologists [5].

Slowly dissolving sutures

Slow-dissolving sutures are useful for fascial closure and intestinal anastomoses, where several weeks of tissue apposition is optimal during healing.

Polydioxanone (PDS II, Ethicon) Polydioxanone is a monofilament suture that retains 74% of its tensile strength at two weeks, 58% at four weeks, and 41% at six weeks. It is stiff and has poor handling and knot-tying properties but causes minimal tissue reaction. Complete hydrolysis occurs after 180-210 days.

Polytrimethylene carbonate (Maxon, Covidien) Polytrimethylene monofilament suture has a high initial tensile strength, higher tensile strength, and greater knot strength than polydioxanone [5]. It retains 81% of its strength at two weeks, 59% at four weeks, and 30% at six weeks. It is wholly hydrolyzed after 180-210 days. Its tissue reactivity is low.

Braided versus monofilament

Braided suture, having higher friction than monofilament, can be secured with fewer throws than monofilament. Its ability to grip tissue makes it popular for ligating vessels and apposing tissue in laparoscopic and arthroscopic surgery. However, it is less resistant to infection, as bacteria can live in the interstices [12]. It also causes more tissue damage during the tying down, as it saws through tissue similar to the wire camping or Gigli saw.

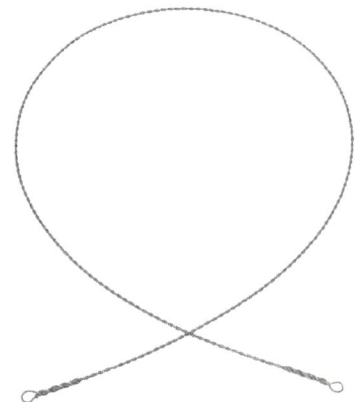

Chapter 3: The Physics of Knots

All knots work by friction and stiffness. Friction occurs from the pressure of the suture against itself and the pressure of the suture against underlying tissue [13]. Stiffness helps prevent slippage at tight turns. Only recently has experimental testing of mathematical formulas been used to study knot security [14], and this has only been done for simple knots [15].

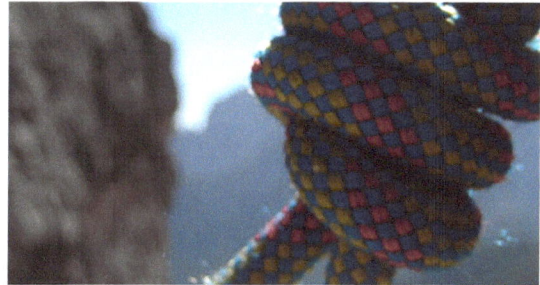

Forget Dark Energy: MIT Physicists Have Finally Cracked Overhand Knots

September 10, 2015//06:30 AM EST

Written by
MICHAEL BYRNE
EDITOR

Mechanical advantage of knot tying

The pulley effect

All knots have a mechanical advantage. In physics, this is described as a pulley or lever effect. The force exerted on tissue is greater than those exerted by your hands. The mechanical advantage is even more significant in knots with a double loop around the tissue (such as the Constrictor knot).

Mechanical advantages in tissue constriction or apposition:

The advantage of pulley from second turn assumes minimal friction of suture with material (like monofilament suture).

The capstan effect would reduce mechanical advantages somewhat due to friction of the suture on the tissue

● Fixed pulley
● Unfixed pulley

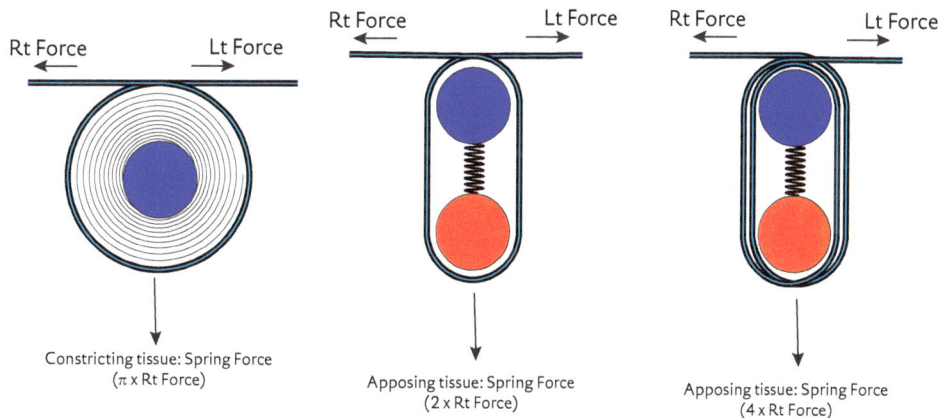

Rt Force   Lt Force

Constricting tissue: Spring Force
(π x Rt Force)

Rt Force   Lt Force

Apposing tissue: Spring Force
(2 x Rt Force)

Rt Force   Lt Force

Apposing tissue: Spring Force
(4 x Rt Force)

Suture friction

Friction occurs between loops of suture and between the suture and tissue. Braided suture generally has a higher friction coefficient than monofilament suture, aiding in knot security, but it can saw through tissue. Thinner suture cuts through fat, preventing it from falling off a pedicle but increasing its risk for breakage. The formula for frictional force is the frictional coefficient multiplied by the force perpendicular to the surface (normal force). It does not depend on the surface contact area when contact does not curve around an object.

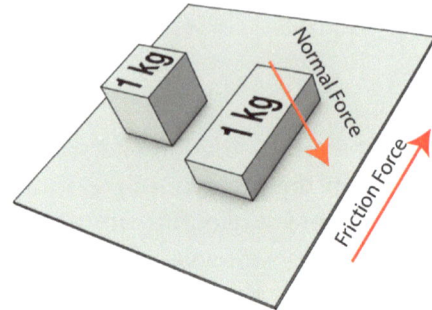

$$Friction = \mu \times Force_{normal}$$

The frictional coefficient of nylon on nylon is 0.15 - 0.25, polyethylene on polyethylene is 0.2 and silk on silk is 0.25 [16].

Chirality

When a suture bends and does not remain on a single plane, it has a property called chirality. This is frequently referred to as "handedness". A 360-degree loop can either have right ("Z") or left ("S") chirality. To determine if your suture follows right or left chirality, hold your right hand in front of you, point your thumb up and curl your fingers. If the suture is in the direction of your fingers, you have a right chirality twist. If the suture loop doesn't match the curl of your fingers, then it has left chirality.

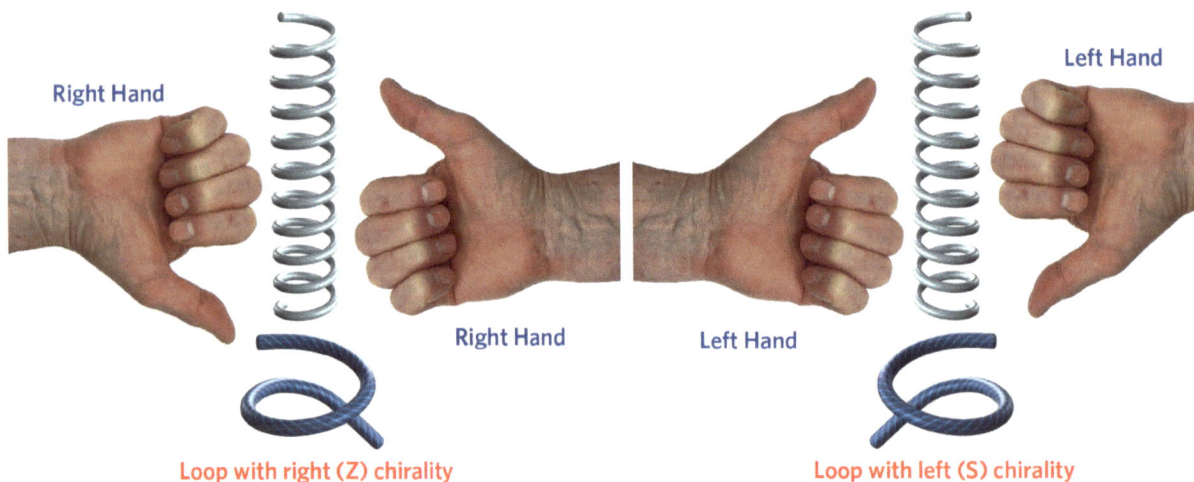

Right Hand   Right Hand   Left Hand   Left Hand

Loop with right (Z) chirality   Loop with left (S) chirality

A clove hitch has two adjacent loops with the same chirality, either both Z or both S.

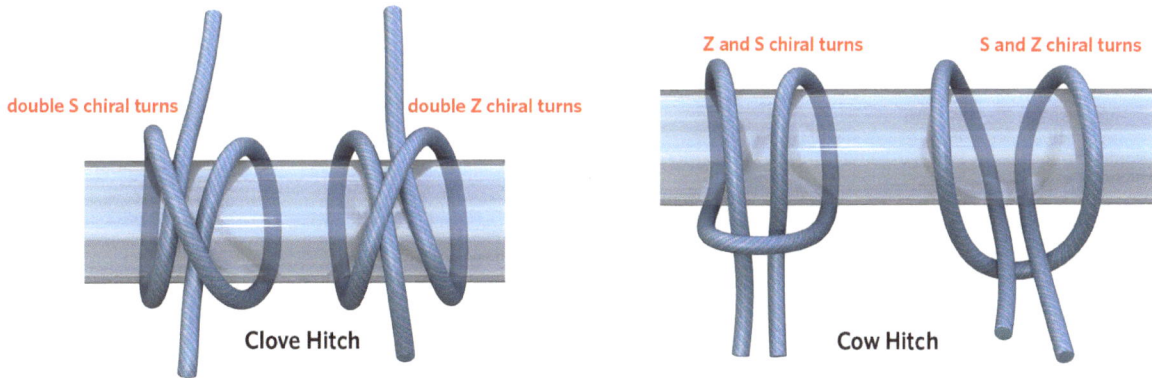

double S chiral turns   double Z chiral turns   Z and S chiral turns   S and Z chiral turns

Clove Hitch   **Cow Hitch**

In contrast, a cow hitch has two adjacent loops with opposite chirality. When two adjacent loops have the same chirality, the frictional force is stronger than if they have opposite chirality. Loops with the same chirality grip more securely and are less likely to slip.

Capstan effect

The hold-force to the load-force of a flexible cord wound around a cylinder is given by the capstan formula [17, 18], which shows that a small holding force exerted on one side can carry a much larger loading force on the other side. The difference in forces is exponentially related to the angle that the cord wraps around the cylinder and the coefficient of friction.

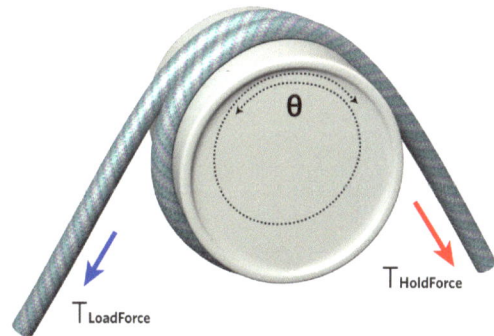

$$T_{load} = T_{hold}e^{\mu\theta}$$

This formula can be derived as follows [19]:

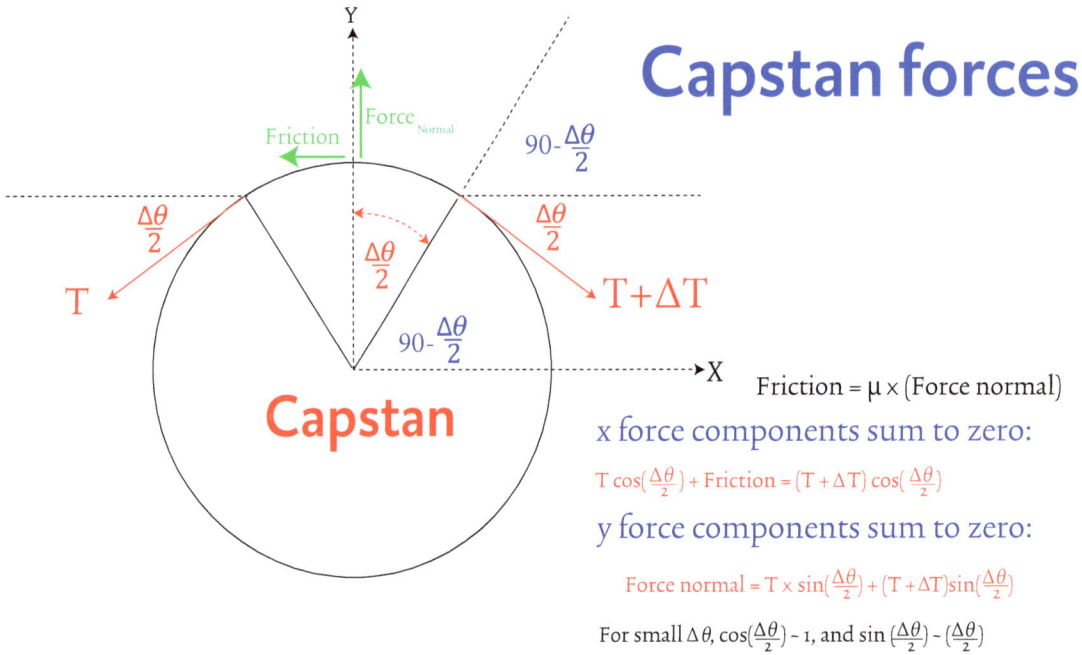

Capstan forces

Friction = $\mu \times$ (Force normal)

x force components sum to zero:

$T\cos(\frac{\Delta\theta}{2}) + \text{Friction} = (T + \Delta T)\cos(\frac{\Delta\theta}{2})$

y force components sum to zero:

$\text{Force normal} = T \times \sin(\frac{\Delta\theta}{2}) + (T + \Delta T)\sin(\frac{\Delta\theta}{2})$

For small $\Delta\theta$, $\cos(\frac{\Delta\theta}{2}) \sim 1$, and $\sin(\frac{\Delta\theta}{2}) \sim (\frac{\Delta\theta}{2})$

Based on the approximation, the x force components can be simplified to T + Friction = (T + Δ T), or Friction = ΔT. The y force components can be simplified to Force normal = T × $\Delta\theta$.
Since Frictional force = μ × (Force normal) and μ × (Force normal) = ΔT, then μ × T × $\Delta\theta$ = ΔT.
When one takes the limit as $\Delta\theta$ approaches 0, the formula simplifies to

$$\frac{dT}{d\theta} = \mu T \qquad \text{or} \qquad \frac{dT}{T} = \mu \, d\theta \qquad \int_{T_{hold}}^{T_{load}} \frac{dT}{T} = \int_{0}^{\theta} \mu \, d\theta$$

$$\text{so} \qquad \ln(T_{load} - T_{hold}) = \mu\theta \qquad \text{or} \qquad T_{load} = T_{hold}\,e^{\mu\theta}$$

When a loop crosses over itself - termed a "riding turn" - the capstan effect becomes important. The loop will exert force on the underlying suture at the point of crossing. If the free end is pulled just to the point of slippage, the force pulling will be equal and opposite to the frictional force of the suture.

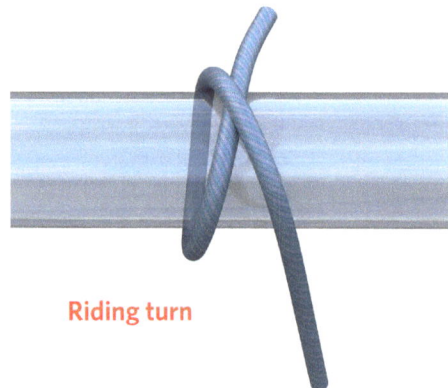

Riding turn

$$T_{load} = \mu \times N, \text{ but also, } T_{load} = T_{hold} \times e^{\mu\theta}$$

The hold force will be the same regardless of the number of wraps, assuming that only the first wrap is crossed and the hold force is just what prevents that loop from sliding. The normal (compressive) force for one wrap would be:

$$N = T_{hold} \frac{e^{\mu\theta}}{\mu}$$

Since one turn is 2π radians, $N = T_{hold} \frac{e^{2\mu\pi}}{\mu}$

The normal force for more than one wrap would be

$$N = T_{hold} \frac{e^{2\mu\pi \times turns}}{\mu}$$

Each additional turn will increase the normal force by a factor of $e^{2\pi\mu}$. Most common plastic-type materials have coefficients of friction between 0.1 and 0.2 [16], so going from one to two turns would increase friction by at least 80%, calculated from friction coefficient of 0.1 [17].

The physics is somewhat more complicated, as stiffness, deformation and indenting, stretch, and friction of the suture with itself will be additional factors. Still, these are generally less significant than the capstan effect itself.

Suture stiffness

The capstan equation ignores stiffness, though modifications of the formula with experimental data have recently been published [20]. Tight turns resist slippage due to stiffness in the suture [14]. This can be seen by the locking that occurs with a single half hitch if you pull up hard on both ends of a suture, and it is a reason to avoid pulling both ends of a suture hard upwards during knot tying.

Suture breakage

All knots reduce the strength of the suture [21, 22]. Knots with minimal bends, like the Clove Hitch, reduce suture strength by about 25%. Like the Square knot, knots with tight loops reduce suture strength by about 55%. If there is asymmetrical tension on a knot, such as in the case of a continuous suture, flat knots are more likely to break than a noose [23, 24].

Tight bends cause stretch on the outside of the curve in the suture and compress the inside of the curve. Due to the tearing force on the outside bend, monofilament sutures will have higher stiffness and a greater tendency to break around tight bends than braided sutures. Even with braided rope, studies from climbing ropes show that if a knot is cinched down into a radius turn smaller than twice its diameter, it gets weakened. (A Figure-eight knot, which has wider loops than a Bowline knot, weakens rope by about 20%, while the tighter loop in a Bowline weakens rope by around 50%.) The frictional force may weaken the suture as friction increases in the contact regions with tight curvature (related to the Capstan effect).

Knot security

After pulling down the first throw, there is back slippage in all knots. Primary security (efficiency to reduce slippage for the final knot compared to the first throw) = final retained load (E1)/load under tension (E2).

Total primary slippage of the ligature = E1 / E2. Data from Howard Taylor [25] is given below:

	Polypropylene	Polyglactin	Polydioxanone	Polyglecaprone
Constrictor	30%	18%	38%	29%
Surgeon's	3%	1%	9%	2%
Modified Surgeon's	15%	6%	22%	18%
SDOS	10%	10%	22%	12%
Strangle	4%	3%	4%	10%
Modified Miller's	2%	3%	2%	5%

A second turn can also improve security. For the Surgeon's knot, a second turn results in a 2-9 fold improvement, depending on the suture material. Secondary security depends on shock or cyclical loading, the stretch of the suture material over time, and whether additional flat knots are added to reduce slippage in response to repeated stresses.

Importance of physics for the surgeon

The choice of suture will affect surgical strength and knot security. Sutures with low friction coefficients are less likely to saw through tissue, but they will generally be stiffer and more difficult to tie securely. Maintaining tension on both ends of the suture in an upward direction away from the tissue may tear small blood vessels due to the mechanical forces generated. Tight turns in knots weaken the suture significantly, accounting for most suture breakage from biomechanical forces occurring at the site of a knot.

The first throw of a Surgeon's knot may be more resistant to slipping than the first throw of a Square knot (known as an Overhand knot), but it will require more tension to tie down, increasing the risk of breaking or being too loose. This is due to the Capstan effect, since an overhand knot has one complete revolution of the suture around itself, whereas the first throw of a Surgeon's knot has two full revolutions. Assuming a frictional coefficient of 0.1, to get the same tension at the halfway point in a Square knot (one-half revolution) compared with a Surgeon's knot (one revolution), you will have to exert about 37% more force on each end.

When a Square knot is converted to a noose, the wrap within the noose will form a Cow Hitch. In contrast, when a Granny knot is converted to a noose, the wrap within the noose will form a Clove Hitch. The frictional forces of the wrap within the noose will be greater in the Granny noose than in the Square noose since a Clove Hitch has two wraps in the same direction where the forces are exponential. In contrast, a Cow Hitch has two wraps in opposite directions where the forces are additive. Assuming a coefficient of friction of 0.1, a Granny noose grips the post part of the suture about 44% more than a Square noose.

Chapter 4: Common Knots

Tying techniques for surgery originated at a time when suture was thicker and composed of materials like catgut, silk, and cotton. These sutures had high friction when tied and generated more inflammation and scarring compared with modern sutures. The Square knot and Surgeon's knot were reliable for tying sutures down. Although suture materials have changed, tying techniques are often taught based on traditions that worked for older suture materials.

Flat knots

Square knot

The Square knot (also known as Reef knot) is the most used knot in surgery. Note that both strands of the suture go either in front of or behind the side loops. This assures that the knot will lie flat and minimizes slippage.

A Square knot can be tied using one-handed or two-handed techniques or with an instrument.

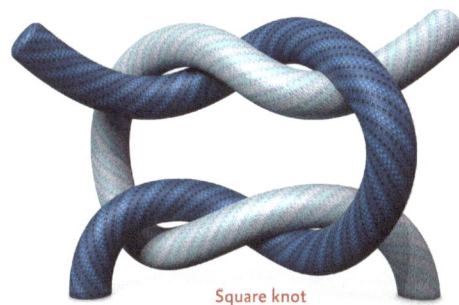

Square knot

Granny knot

The Granny knot differs from the Square knot in that the suture goes in different directions (one in front, one behind) with respect to the side loops, and this rotation of the top throw prevents the knot from lying flat. This makes it more prone to slippage, particularly with cyclical loading.

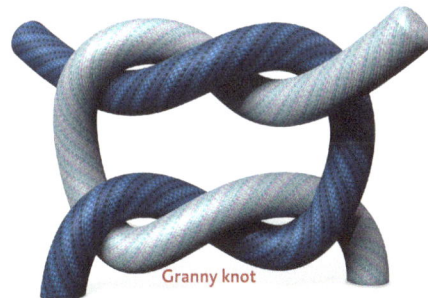

Granny knot

In experimental studies, if tied down firmly, the Granny knot holds about as well as a Square knot [26]. However, unlike a Square knot, it will not self-tighten in response to tension (see **https://vimeo.com/220889855**). Since it is simpler to tie than a Square knot, a Granny knot is sometimes tied inadvertently. Apparently, even a gorilla can tie this knot [27].

Flat knots with reversed chirality, like the Square knot, are more secure than flat knots with the same chirality, like the Granny knot. This was recently demonstrated in a paper from MIT where color-changing photonic fibers were used to image the strain of knots. They showed that simple topological counting rules could predict the relative mechanical stability of knots [28].

While the Square knot is more secure than a Granny if tied flat, the Granny is more secure than the Square Knot when used as a noose. Dr. C. W. Mayo of the Mayo clinic suggested it for ligation of the cystic duct and large vessels when followed by a Square knot to lock it in place [29].

One can tie a Granny knot using one-handed or two-handed techniques by repeating the first part of the throw for the second throw (steps 1-5 one-handed, steps 1-4 two-handed).

Surgeon's knot

Like the Square knot, the Surgeon's knot lies flat, and sutures go in the same direction with respect to each side of the loop (behind or in front).

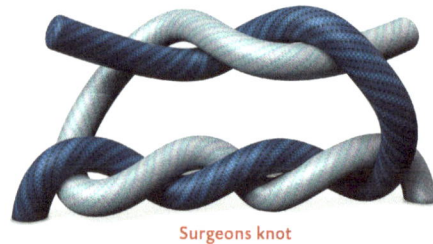

Surgeons knot

The extra coil around the suture in the first throw increases friction and was thought to reduce slippage. This makes the knot less likely to loosen when tying but more difficult to tie tightly [30, 31]. It also increases the possibility of breaking the suture when tying it down tightly [32].

In actual experimental studies, it was not found to be any more secure or less likely to slip than a Square knot when two additional squared throws are added, even with monofilament suture [33].

Comparison of flat knots

The ideal surgical knot will tie a blood vessel securely and appose tissue closely. It will resist untying, breaking, and slipping. It should be simple, easily tied, secure, and not weaken the suture. A combination of slipping knots and adding additional flat throws accomplishes both good apposition of tissue and knot security. Slippage or unraveling places knot security at risk and has been reported to occur in 30-100% of surgical knots [1]. Up to 80% of experienced surgeons do not reliably square down their knots [34].

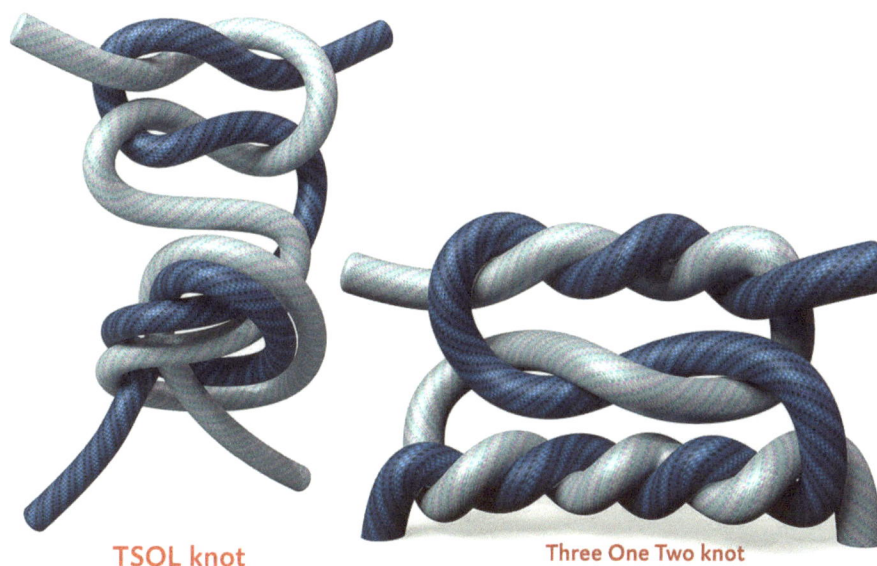

TSOL knot   Three One Two knot

Some knots slip less than Square knots, such as the triple Surgeon's knot [35], the similar 3-1-2 knot [36], and the Mayo Clinic TSOL knot, but these knots are difficult to tie down tightly. The TSOL knot is similar to the Overhand knot used to tie two ropes together for rappelling (sometimes called the European Death knot [37]) but adds a Square knot on top to prevent loosening by knot creep. In the instructional videos from Mayo Clinic, the authors use a pickup or hemostat within the overhand loop to help push this down to prevent poor approximation of tissue edges.

In comparing knot holding strength using PDS monofilament suture, the TSOL knot had over twice the holding strength compared with a four-throw Square knot [1]. TSOL knots failed by suture rupture at 76% of the breaking strength of PDS suture. In contrast, four-throw Square knots generally fail by slippage and untying. However, when tissue is under tension, an instrument is required to push the TSOL knot down. It is difficult to tighten the knot, and it cannot be further tightened after it has been pulled down.

Nooses

Nooses are helpful when it is difficult to tie knots down flat, such as shoulder arthroscopy or gynecological procedures where vascular pedicles are ligated deep in the pelvis [38]. They are also helpful when tying monofilament sutures under tension, as they can be used to ensure that the initial throws do not loosen during tying. They are preferable to Square knots when a continuous running suture is used, as they are less prone to breakage [23, 24]. They are commonly used in shoulder arthroscopy as extracorporeal knots to ensure good tissue apposition. With a noose, tension should be on the sliding side only: pulling on the other side locks the knot. Note that if a knot is tied as a noose rather than individual half hitches, which are pushed down, the non-slipped side will not lengthen as the noose is tightened. This may result in a short suture which is challenging to tie.

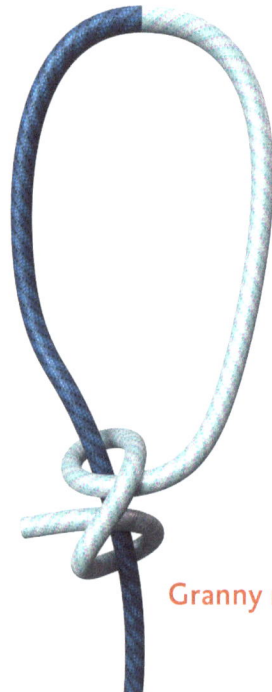

Granny noose

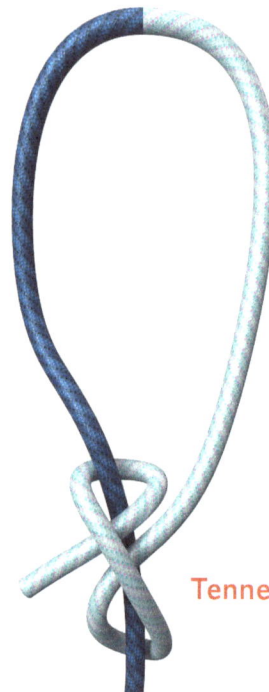

Tennesee Slider

The Granny noose [24] and Tennessee Slider [39–41] slide down as a Clove Hitch, whereas the Square noose [24] forms a Cow's Hitch, making it less secure. Measuring the slippage force for paracord using a tensiometer with a Square and a Granny noose - each tightened to 30 N - the Granny noose required more than twice the force to slip compared with the Square noose (personal test).

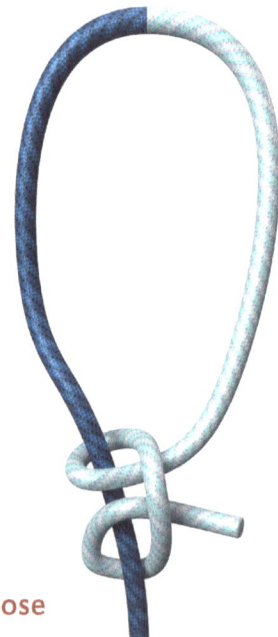

Square noose

The Nicky knot [39–41], which is based on the Taut-line Hitch, is more secure than a Tennessee Slider but slightly more difficult to tie down tightly and more prone to premature locking. It is tied by forming a Surgeon's first throw and a Granny's second throw.

All nooses are at risk for loosening, as the force to slip after they are tied is less than a third of that needed to loosen a knot tied flat [26]. Back slippage can be prevented by throwing half hitches off the other end of the suture for one or two throws after tying down the noose [4]. The Nicky knot, Tennessee Slider, and Roeder knot are not secure unless three reversing half hitches on alternating posts are added to prevent back slipping [40].

An example of sliding off alternating posts is the Revo knot, commonly used in arthroscopic surgery. This knot has been shown to result in tighter loops than hand-tied squared knots and has similar knot security [42].

The Revo knot [39, 40, 42, 43] is tied as two Granny nooses followed by a Square noose, where the first throw of the Square is wrapped around the short end and the second around the long end. It is an effective and secure knot for ligating blood vessels in deep areas [44].

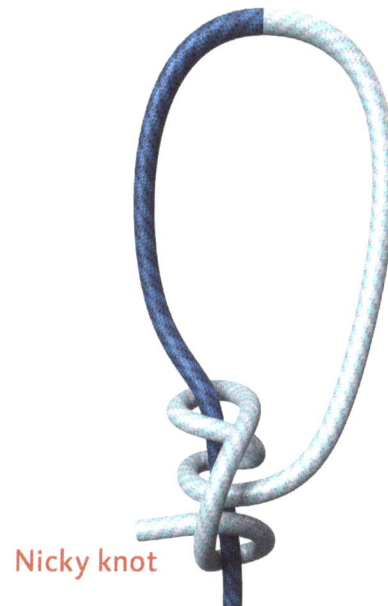

Nicky knot

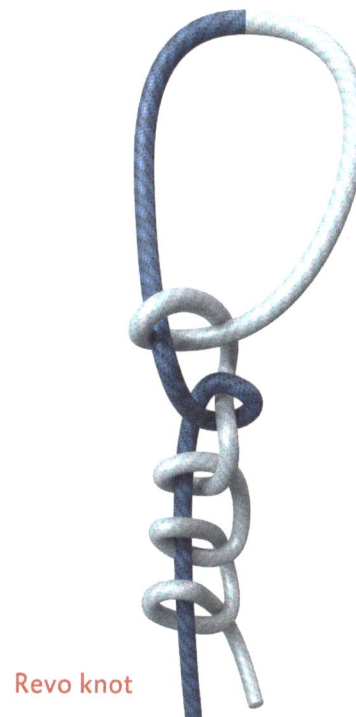

Revo knot

Even more secure than the Tennessee Slider, sliding Granny, and Nicky knots are the similar Roeder and Melzer knots. They are commonly used in laparoscopic surgery as an extracorporeal tie. The Roeder knot [39–41, 45, 46] was first described for tonsillectomies where catgut was used. It was introduced into laparoscopic surgery in 1978. However, when monofilament suture such as PDS is used, the Melzer [39, 40, 45] is more secure than the Roeder knot. Its resistance to slippage is reduced with a larger diameter suture and is doubled for 0-PDS suture compared with 2-0 PDS suture. However, while the Melzer knot has good reliability for monofilament sutures, neither the Roeder nor Melzer knots are reliable for braided material.

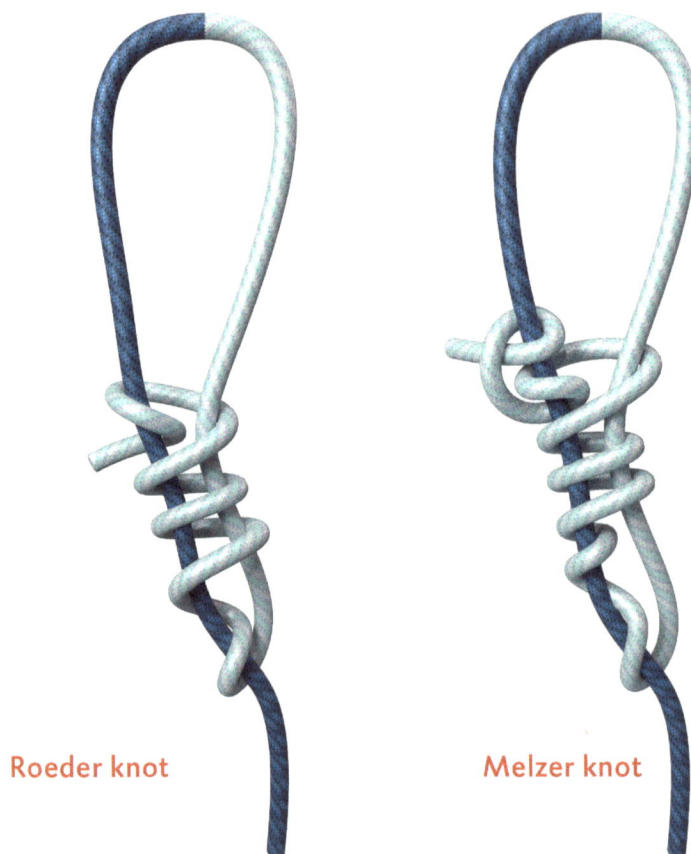

Roeder knot   Melzer knot

Compared to the Roeder, the Melzer knot starts with an extra throw, like a Surgeon's knot, and ends with a second half-hitch.

Tying knots down tightly

Knots should be tied to hold the tissue in good apposition, neither overly tight nor overly loose, not weakening the suture, and not coming untied.

If there is a gap between two pieces of tissue tied with a knot, the entire connection will rely on the strength of the suture rather than on the in-growth of the two sides. This often results in the suture breaking or cutting through the tissue. Conversely, too tight a suture may cause ischemia, resulting in tissue dying and the suture failing to keep edges apposed. The knot should be tied to ensure it lies flat and does not back-slip during the process of tying.

The most common methods to ensure that a knot does not back-slip are:

· Maintain tension on the two strands during tying so that the first throw does not slip.

· Tie the first throw with extra loops so that the friction of the tissue reduces back slippage (examples: Surgeon's knot and 3-1-2 knot).

· Tie down a noose that partially locks in place, preventing back slippage until subsequent security throws are added.

The myth of "maintaining tension" while tying a knot

A single Overhand knot will back-slip if there is tension on the tissue being tied, especially if the suture is monofilament and slippery. A commonly taught technique is to keep tension on both ends of the suture throughout the tying process. This causes several problems:

· Upward tension on the two ends of the suture can cause injury and bleeding.

· The suture is more likely to lock prematurely, causing an air knot.

· Unless the tension on the two ends is precisely the same, the knot may tie down as a noose.

Tissue injury

If the suture is around a blood vessel, the upward tension on the two ends can cause tearing and the avulsion of side branches, leading to injury and bleeding. In addition, the friction of the suture against the tissue can act as a camp-saw to cut into the tissue.

Tissue damage from tension:

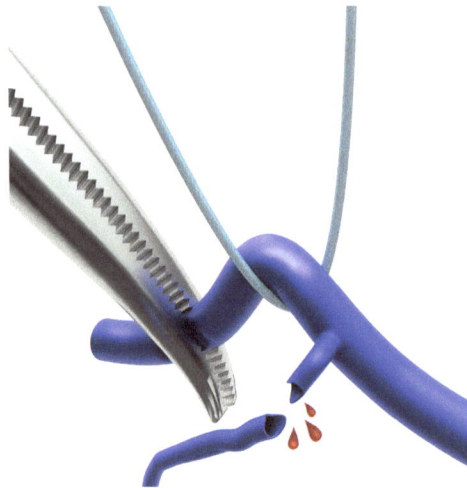

Air Knots

Knots that tie down flat but do not adequately appose tissue or ligate a vessel are called "air knots." When there is a difference in the tension used to pull the two ends of the suture, the overhand first throw can turn into a half hitch. A subsequent throw will lock the knot part down, failing to appose tissue properly.

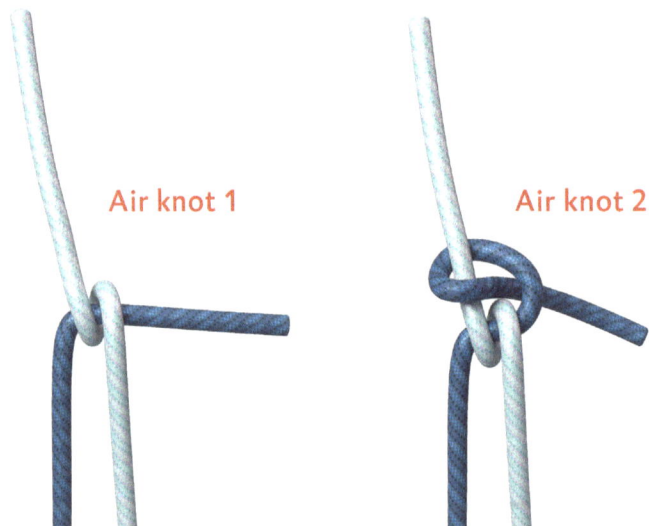

Inadvertent nooses

The knot will not tie down flat unless the tension on the two ends is precisely the same. The side with stronger tension will act as a straight post around which the other side will encircle in a series of half hitches. Even if you pull the short end in opposite directions, you will get a giant noose that is not secure and can slip. This noose cannot be converted back to a flat knot by pulling with equal tension on the two ends of the suture after it is formed.

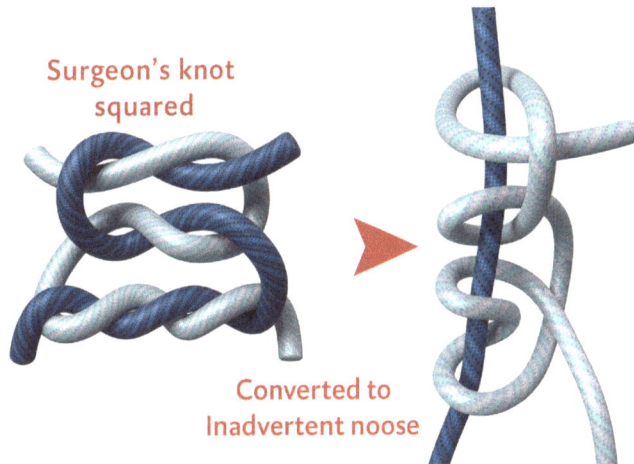

Surgeon's knot squared

Converted to Inadvertent noose

The easiest way to avoid unequal tension is to tie down the knot with no tension, dropping your hands downward as the knot is tightened.

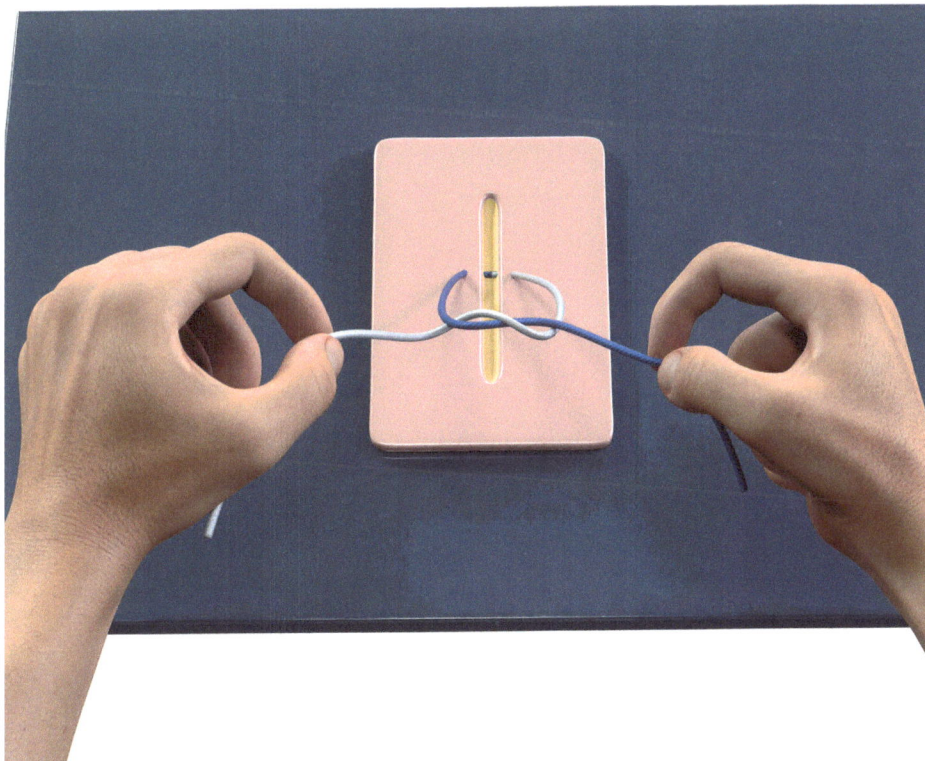

Equal moderate tension itself is difficult to accomplish and slight inequality of tension results in conversion of the flat knot to a noose.

Equal but too much tension

Unequal tension converts to noose

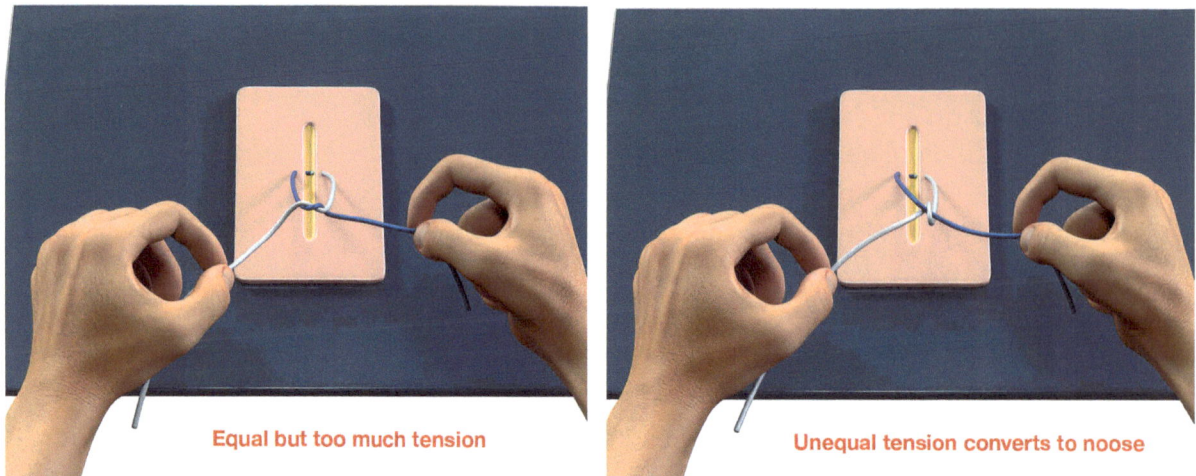

Video showing inadvertent noose due to failure to maintain proper tension: **https://vimeo.com/190935395**

A good example of an inadvertent noose is shown in the award-winning scanning electron micrograph of a surgical suture by Anne Weston [47]. The stitch was removed seven days after suturing a head wound.

Photograph: modified from an image by Anne Weston, EM STP, Francis Crick Institute.

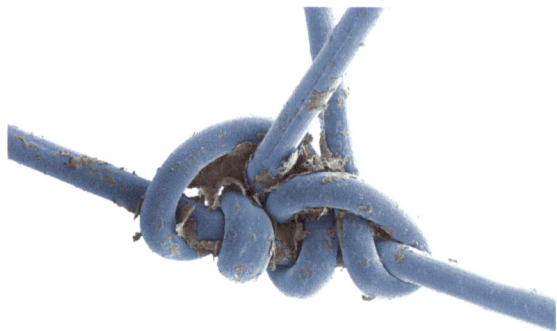

The problem with extra throws on the first knot

A Surgeon's knot has an extra wrap of the two ends of the suture around themselves and adds greater friction between the tissue and the first throw, helping to reduce back-slippage.

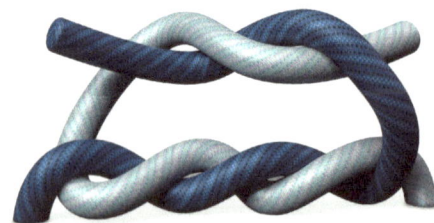

Surgeons knot

Like the Square knot, the Surgeon's knot lies flat, and sutures go out the same direction with respect to each side of the loop (behind or in front). However, the extra coil around the sutures in the first throw increases friction and reduces slippage. This makes the knot less likely to loosen when tying but more challenging to tie tightly [30, 31]. It increases the possibility of breaking the suture when trying to tie it down [32]. It is not any more secure or less likely to slip than a Square knot when two additional squared throws are added, even with monofilament suture [33].

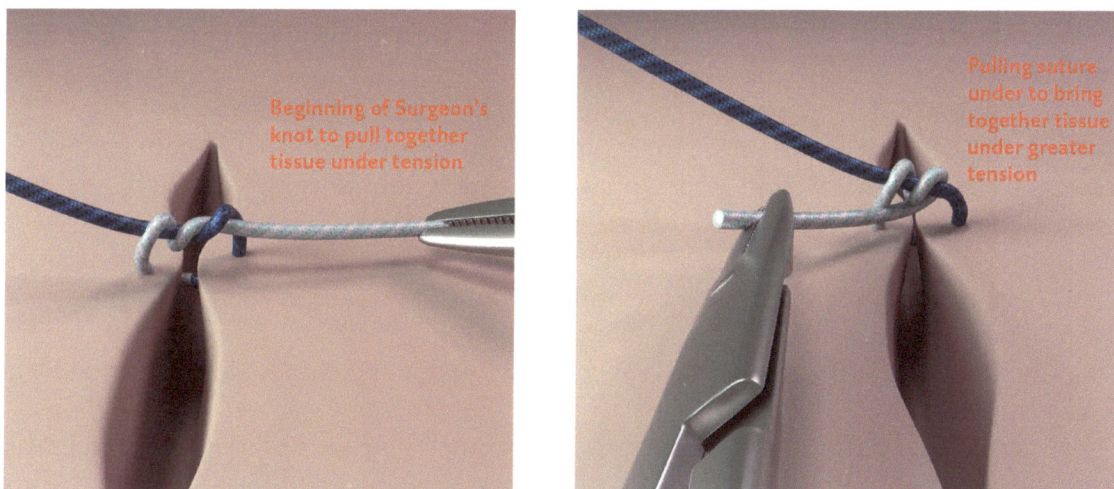

To further reduce slippage, the two ends of the suture can be pulled in the same direction, as is commonly taught with a Surgeon's knot tied as an instrument knot. This sometimes works if the tension on the two sides of the tissue is minimal, but it is unreliable with a monofilament suture if any significant tension exists. Furthermore, adding additional throws significantly increases the tension required to pull the two pieces of tissue together, resulting in an increased chance of a loose initial throw and suture breakage. The 3-1-2 knot has been proposed as having less chance of unraveling than a Surgeon's knot, but its increased friction makes it even more prone to tying down loosely and fracturing the suture. The Mayo Clinic TSOL knot has the advantage of reduced risk for suture breakage but is even harder to tie down tightly.

Video of super-surgeon's knot showing inability to approximate tissue:
https://vimeo.com/190934177

Tying down a noose: pros and cons

Tying a noose for the first two throws is generally a reliable way of tying a knot with good apposition and tension and helps to prevent back slippage. The noose reduces but does not prevent back slippage, and it is necessary to tie subsequent throws down flat. The number of flat throws to ensure knot security does not count the slipped portions, so the knot itself is often bulkier.

A noose cannot be converted back to a flat knot after it has been tied down, even by pulling the strands in opposite directions.

The least reliable noose is a Square knot that has been converted into a noose. The portion of the suture that wraps around the straight post is a Cow Hitch. This knot has almost twice the likelihood of back slipping compared with the Granny noose, which wraps around the straight post as a Clove Hitch.

Complex nooses and locking knots have greater security than a Square or Granny noose. They are instrumental in arthroscopic surgery or for tying a knot in a deep, hard-to-reach area, where apposition of tissue with the first throw is essential. Information about these knots can be found on page 113, "Locking knots".

Securing the knot

The first stage of tying a knot (the first two throws) is crucial, assuring that the knot adequately secures or apposes tissue. The second stage (subsequent throws) provides knot security by preventing back slippage or untying when the knot is released. As can be seen on page 12, "Knot security", the final tension on a knot is significantly less than when the knot is being tied and there is tension on both ends of the suture. When you let go of the ends of the suture, the forces reverse, and stiffness and friction help to prevent the knot from untying. Security is assured by adding additional throws where the ends are pulled down flat.
Back slippage can also be prevented by slipping down opposite posts. The Revo knot, formed this way, may be the best choice when the only option is to pull the ends of the suture towards and away from the surgeon.

Locking knots are another alternative, but even these can be unreliable without additional security throws.

The Constrictor knot maintains security after tension is released without additional throws. It is reliable for securing blood vessels.

Tying down flat knots

Three factors must be performed to ensure flat knots:

· The knot structure must be correct. Knots should be tied down in a Square, not Granny conformation, to prevent rotation of the knot and slippage.

· The ends of the knot must be pulled down in the correct direction, with each throw rotated 180 degrees to the previous throw.

· Force on the two ends must be equal. Avoid creating a post around which the other end of the suture can wrap. Keep each end loose until the knot goes down flat, and only then give a tug to tighten the knot into position.

Match the knot to the suture

High friction sutures

Silk sutures have high friction, and three squared throws will not slip, even when the ends of the knot are cut short [48].

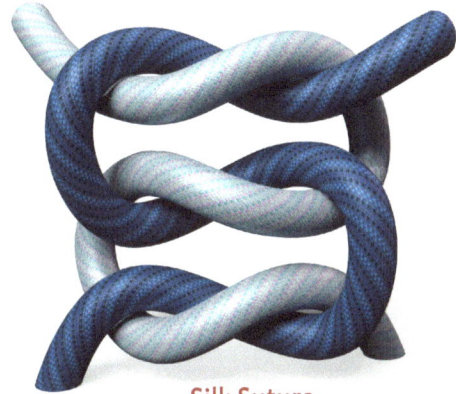

Silk Suture

Medium friction sutures

Dexon and Vicryl (absorbable) and Ethibond (permanent) are braided sutures with moderate friction. They are generally tied with four squared throws, leaving a 1/8-inch tail. The first throw can be done as a Surgeon's knot, either pulled down straight or pulled back on itself to generate additional friction and prevent slippage.

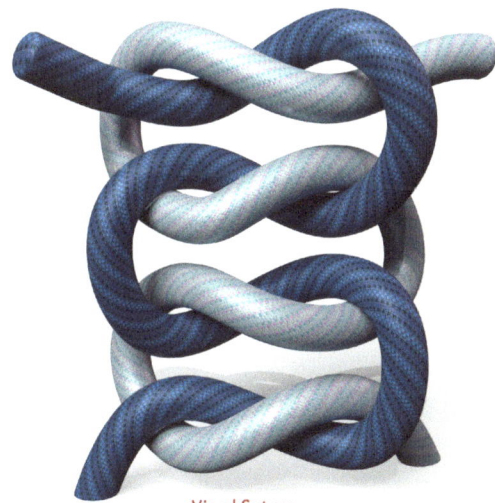

Vicryl Suture

Low friction sutures

Monofilament sutures are widely used because, like fishing line, they have low friction and reduce sawing or cutting of tissue. They are the least reactive and most resistant to infection. However, they are stiff and not ideal for areas where softer sutures are needed for patient comfort. They also require additional throws for security [49].

Examples of permanent monofilament sutures include Ethilon and Prolene. Slowly absorbable monofilament sutures include PDS and Maxon. Fast absorbable sutures used often for subcuticular closure include Monocryl, Biosyn, and Caprosyn. All monofilament sutures except Biosyn tie like fishing line.

Five to seven squared throws are needed to prevent slippage, and leaving at least a 1/8-inch tail is important. Since they have very little friction, Square and Surgeon's knots may result in a loose knot. To avoid this, many use a noose for the first two throws.

The downside to adding multiple squared throws for security is an increased risk for suture extrusion. In a porcine model, using subcuticular knots of 4-o polysorb, the chance of suture extrusion was 30% for five throws, 17% for four throws, and 10% for three throw square knots [50].

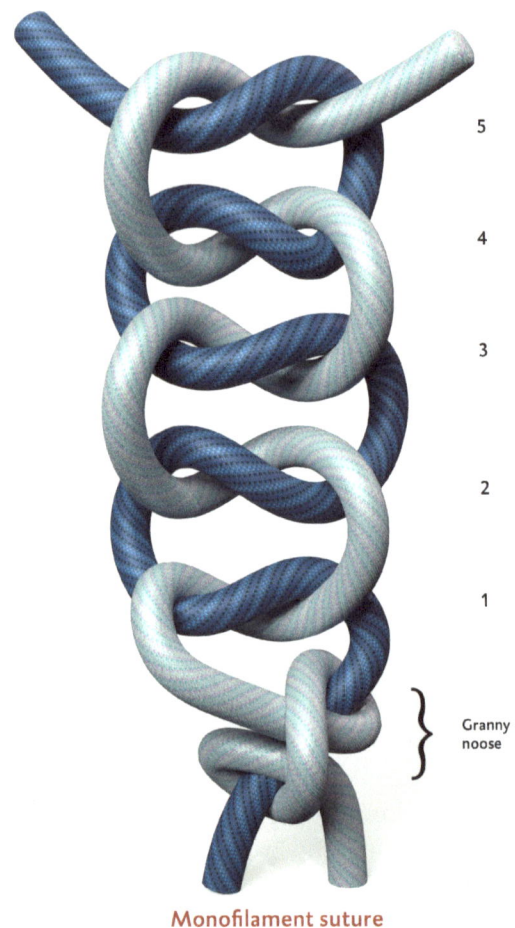

Monofilament suture

Chapter 5: One and Two Hand Ties

Hand ties

The starting position is the same for both one-handed and two-handed ties. If you are right-handed, you should suture forehand, from right to left through tissue. The needle is pulled through the tissue along its natural curve and grasped in a needle holder in the right hand. The needle is then released from the needle driver, and the long end of the suture (with the needle) is held in the right hand with the right palm facing downwards. The easiest way to hold the suture with the right hand is to wrap the suture around the middle part of the right middle finger in multiple overlapping loops, starting an inch or two away from the needle. This allows the suture to be securely held without griping it tightly. You can shorten or lengthen the part of the suture used for the knot by altering the number of wraps of suture around your right middle finger.

Your left hand should hold the short end of the suture between your left thumb and index finger, with your hand held like an "OK" sign and your left palm facing upwards. The short end of the suture should be slightly closer to you than the long end.

You generally suture forehand through tissue from left to right if you are left-handed. For both right-handed and left-handed surgeons, one-hand (or one-handed) knots are tied with the non-dominant hand, and two-hand knots are tied with the dominant hand. The illustrations in this book show the positions of a right-handed surgeon; the correct hand position for a left-handed surgeon would be the mirror image of the illustrations. (see page 38, "What if you are left-handed?")

One-handed Square knot

The term "one-hand knot" or "one-handed knot" is derived from the practice of tying with the non-dominant hand while holding a needle holder in the dominant hand. Holding the needle holder while tying the knot lessens the ability to judge tension between the two ends, so it is best to remove the needle from the needle holder and tie the suture with both hands. Tied correctly, the one-handed knot is simply a way of tying knots using both hands that is more efficient than the two-hand tying method. The hand not doing the tying should bring the other end of the suture towards the tying hand to complete the loop. This reduces unnecessary motion of the tying hand.

One-handed knots pull the suture through with relatively weak intrinsic muscles of the hand. One can easily drop the suture unless they pay attention to the steps where stronger forearm muscles substitute the grip on the suture.

Step 1: Using your right hand and keeping your left palm up, bring the long end of the suture across the palm of your left hand. This is the starting position for both one-hand and two-hand ties. It is helpful to hold the suture between your left thumb and index finger well away from your other fingers.

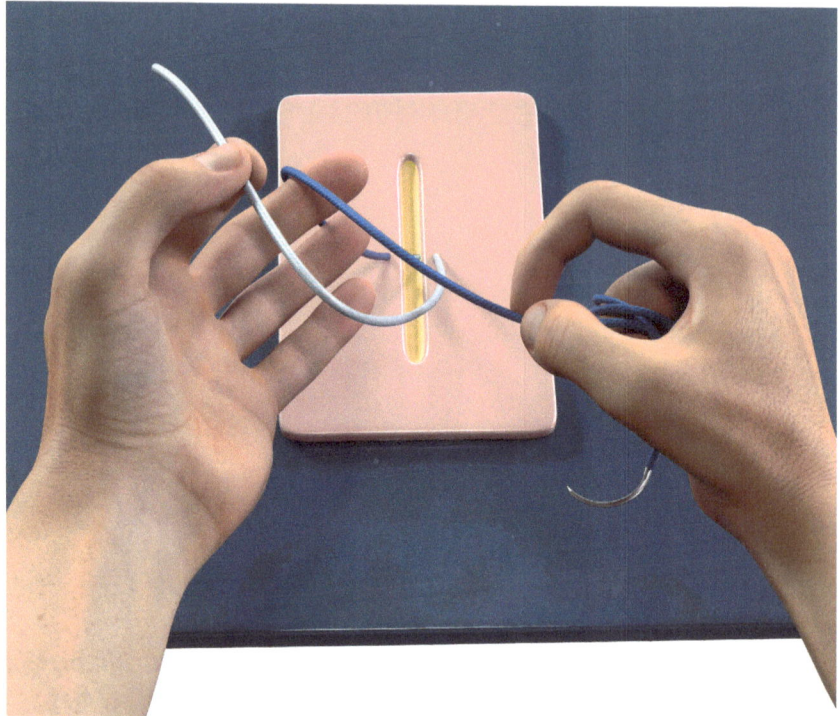

Step 2: Bend your left middle finger under the short end of the suture, preparing to catch the short end of the suture between the back of your left middle finger and front of your left ring finger.

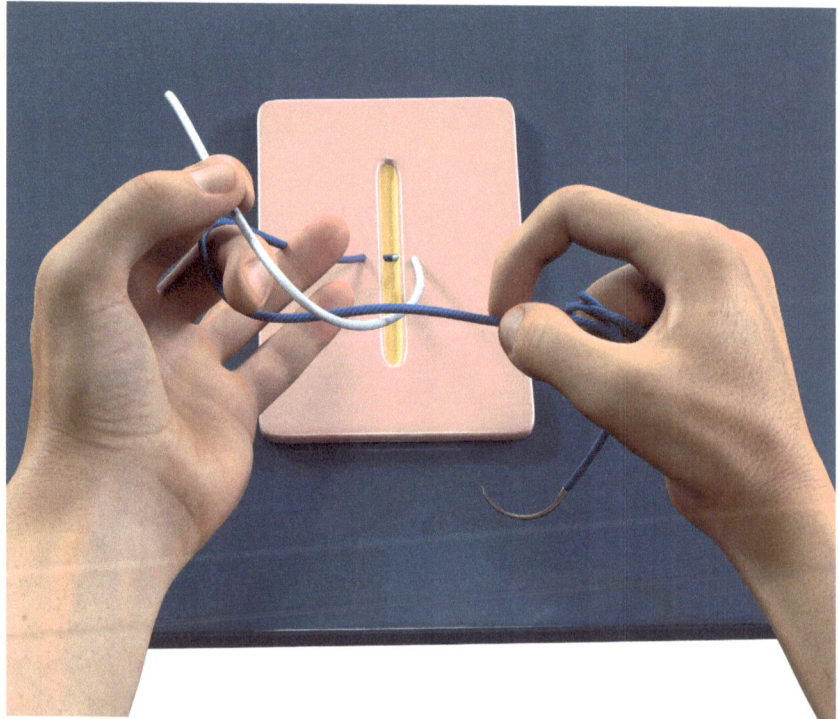

Step 3: Catch the short end of the suture between your left middle and ring finger and release the grip on the suture between your thumb and index finger.

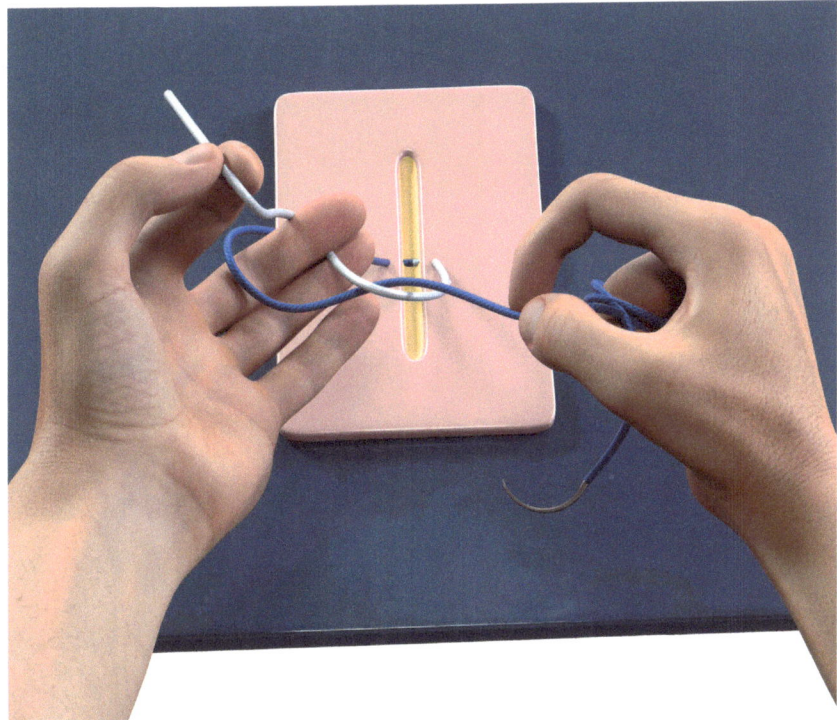

Step 4: Pull the tip of the suture's short end under the suture's long end.

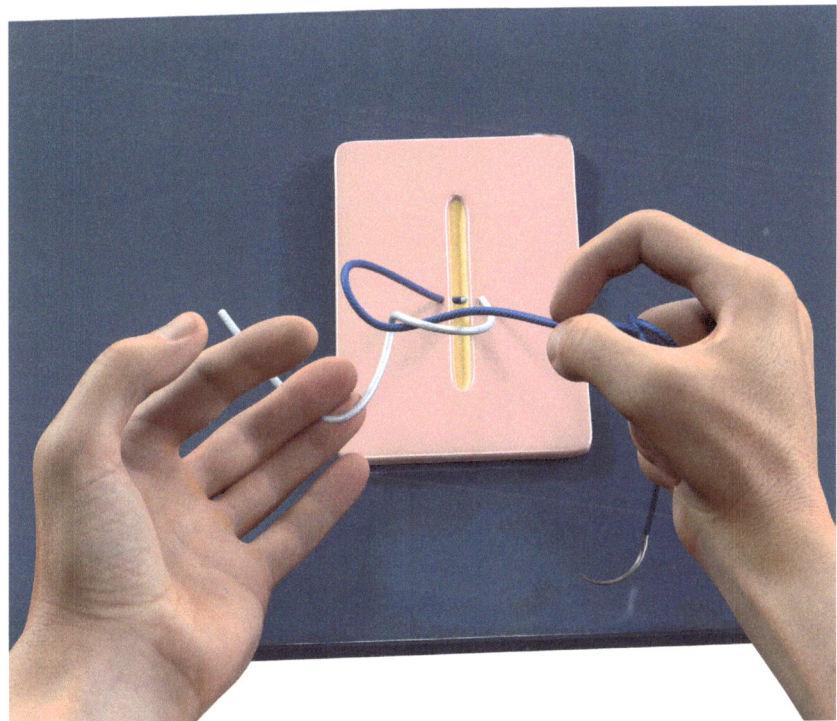

Step 5: Turn your left hand palm down. Grab the short end of the suture between your left thumb and the distal joint of your left middle finger. Use your two index fingers to pull the suture down flat.

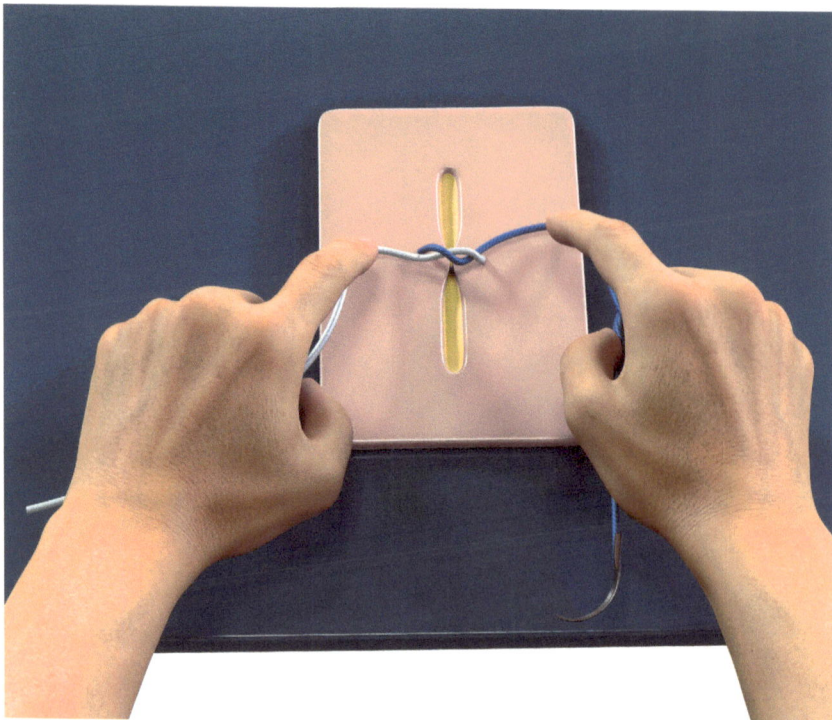

Step 6: Point your left index finger beyond the suture.

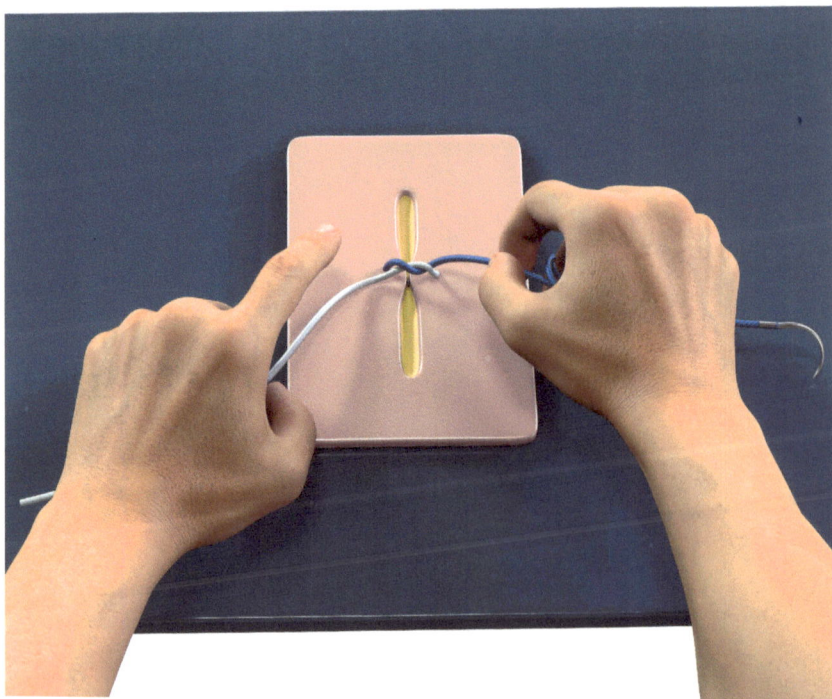

Step 7: Turn your left palm upwards. Your left thumb and palm side of your distal middle finger joint should be holding the suture, and your left index finger should be extended enough to create a space between your index and middle fingers.

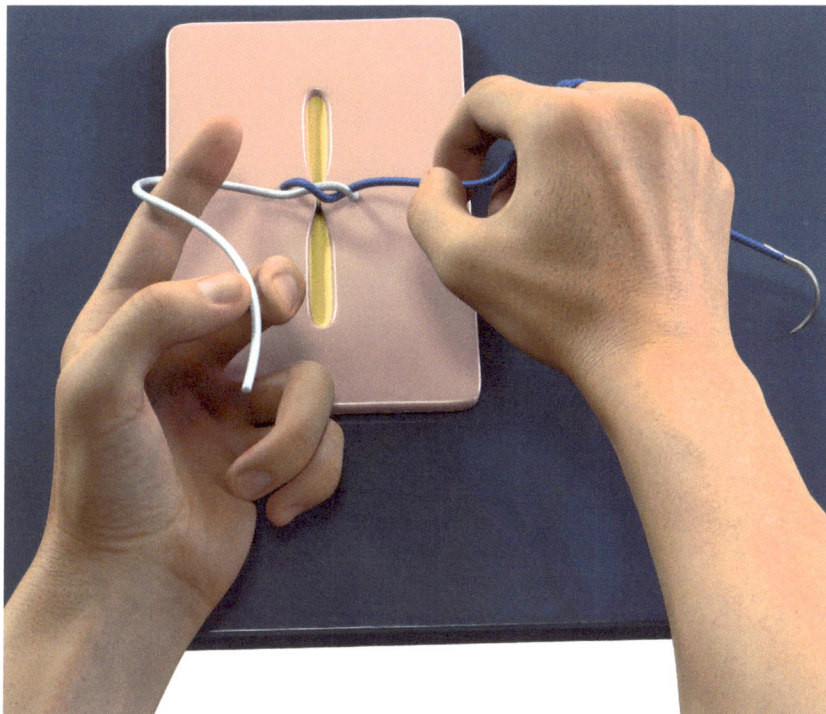

Step 8: Use your right hand to pull the suture across your left index finger to create a loop.

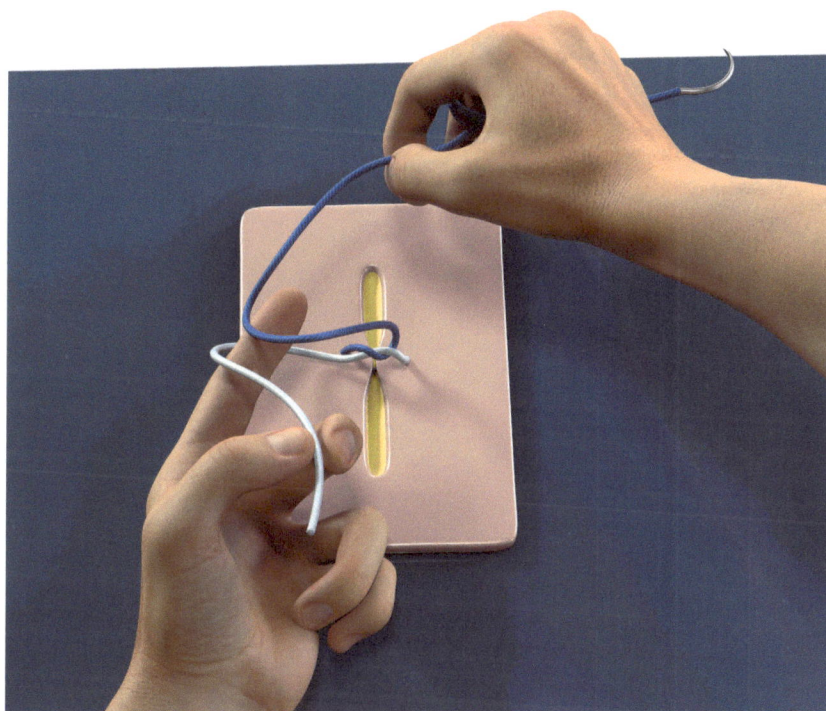

Step 9: Hook your left index finger back under the short end of the suture, pulling the long end with it. This will be made easier if you lower your right hand.

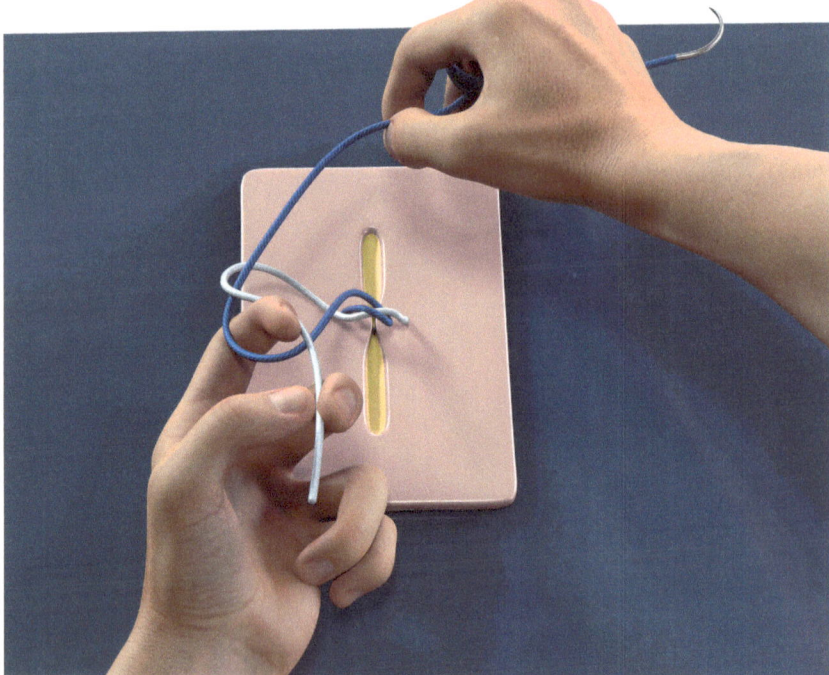

Step 10: Use the back of your left index finger to pull the short end downward.

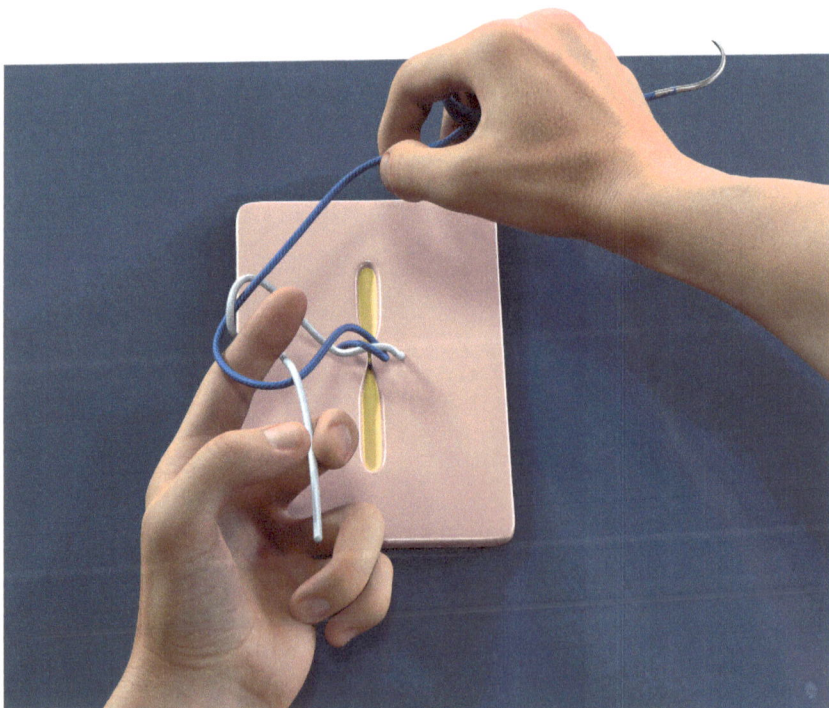

Step 11: Turn your left hand palm down, pulling the short end of the suture under the long end while still gripping the tail of the suture between your left thumb and middle finger.

Note: Students are frequently taught at this point to grip the suture between their left index and middle fingers and to pull the suture through the loop. This is not recommended. The suture is often dropped when doing this, and the weak intrinsic muscles of the hand are inadequate to hold it securely.

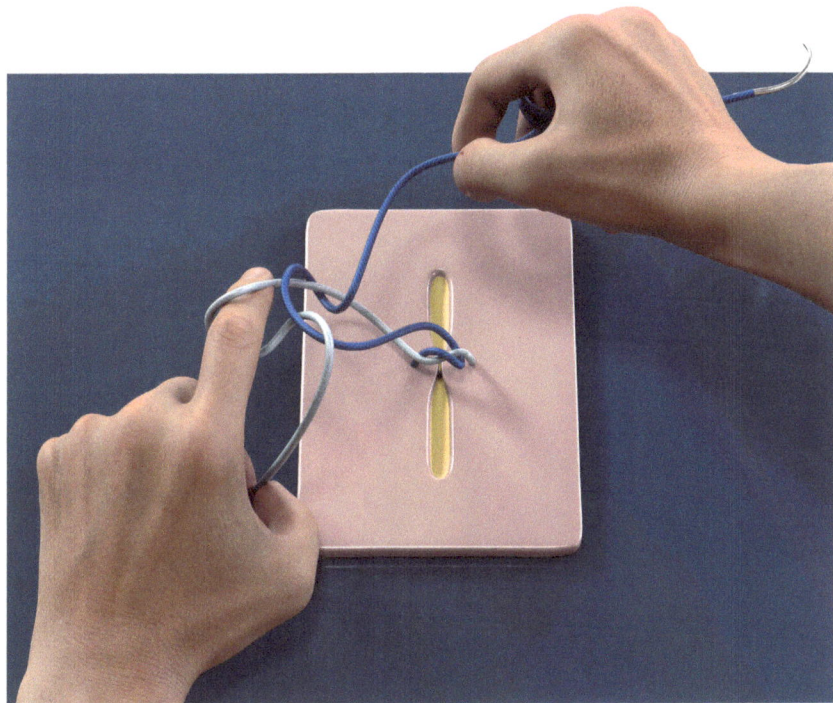

Step 12: Turn your left hand palm up and start flexing your left index finger. Continue flexing your left index finger until it pinches the suture between your index finger and thumb.

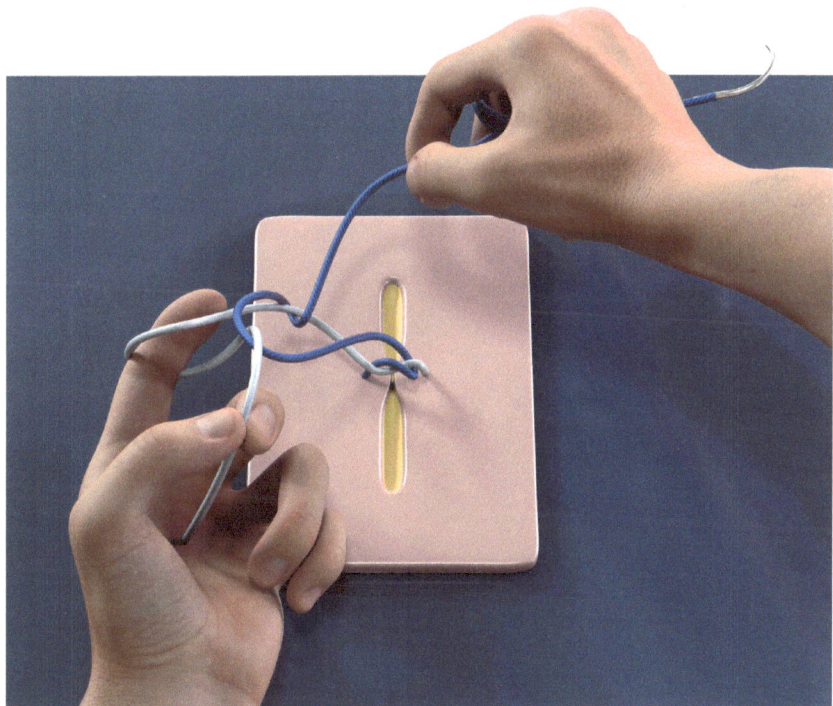

Step 13: Let go of the suture's short end except where it is held between your index finger and thumb.

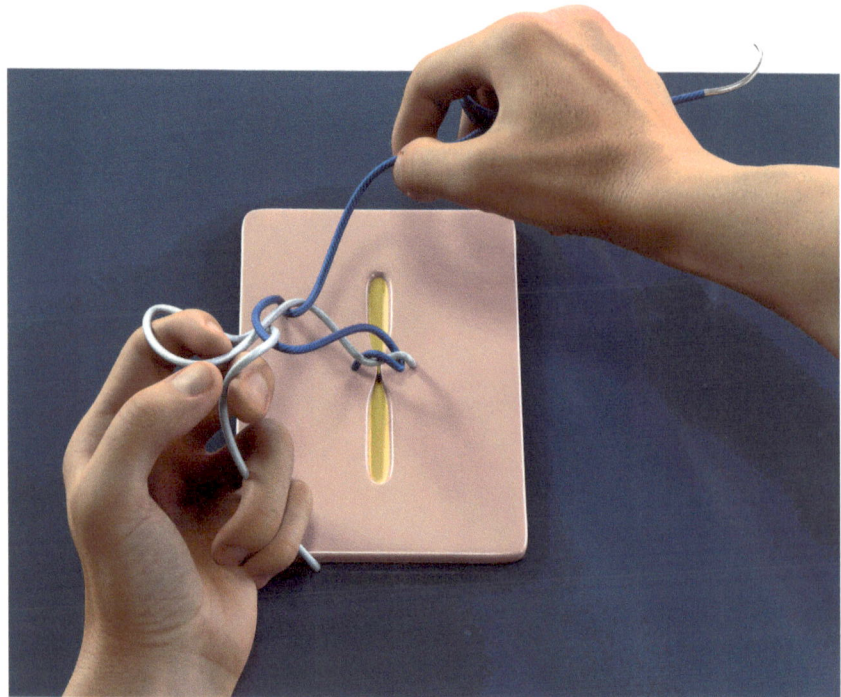

Step 14: Flatten the knot, pushing down on the short end of the suture with your left fourth and fifth fingers, with your left palm facing down. The second knot will lie at right angles to the first. Pull all subsequent knots down flat towards or away from you to avoid crossing your hands.

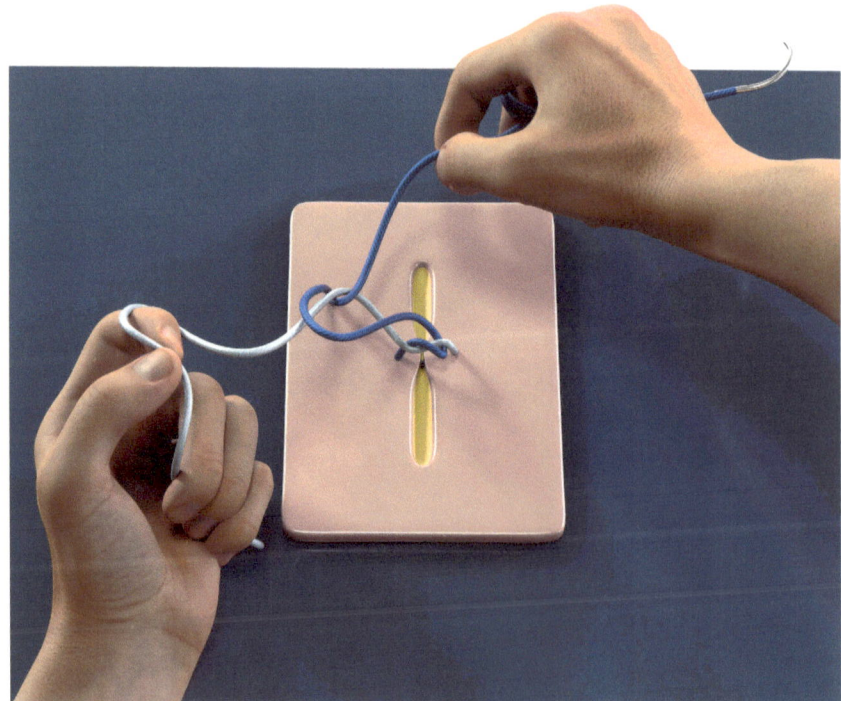

Step 15: Turn your left palm up and pull your right hand towards you to create a loop like you did in step 1. Repeat steps 1-4.

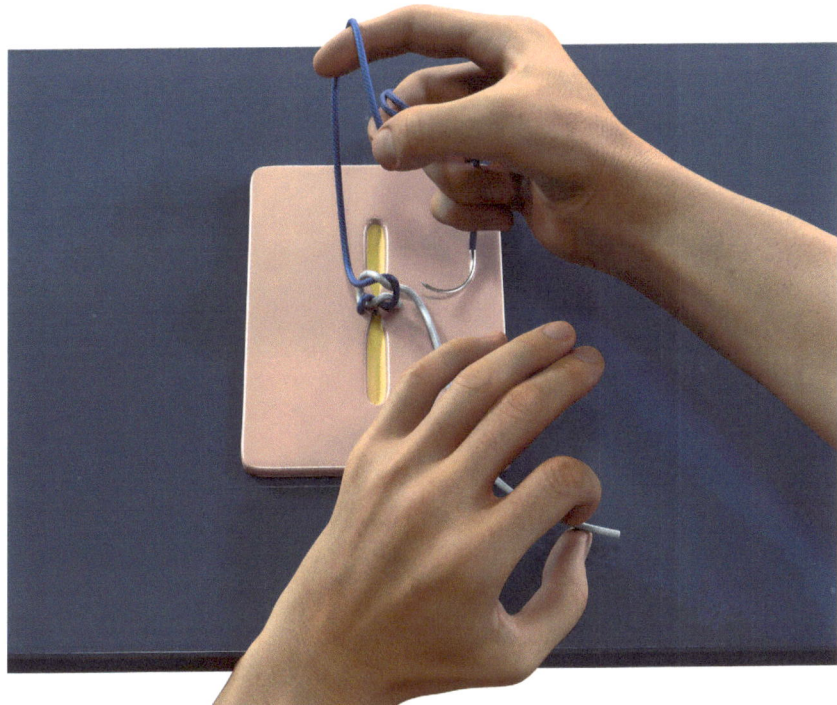

Step 16: Pull the knot down flat by looping the suture under your left index finger. Keeping your left palm up, pull the short end of the suture away from you. If desired, you can rotate your left palm down again to help flatten the knot. Continue tying the knot following steps 7-14.

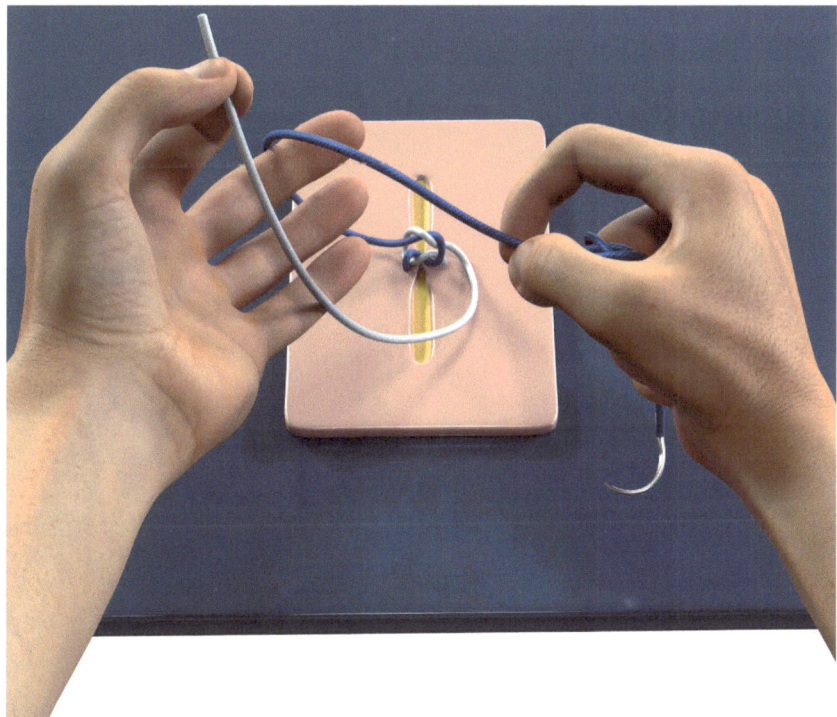

Video of a one-handed tie with slipped Granny knot:
https://vimeo.com/190934562

What if you are left-handed?

Surgeons are more precise when they suture from their dominant side towards their non-dominant side, like a forehand swing in tennis. That means that right-handed people generally suture from their right towards their left. When tying a knot, and the needle end will be towards their left. After crossing the ends so that the knot will come down flat, two-hand ties should be performed with the right hand and one-hand ties with the left hand. This technique prevents pulling the needle end through the loop.

Left-handed surgeons generally suture from their left towards their right. When tying a knot, the needle will start towards their right. Left-handed surgeons should learn to perform two-hand ties with the left hand and one-hand ties with the right hand. The illustrations in this book show the general hand positions of a right-handed surgeon but are mirror images of a left-handed surgeon.

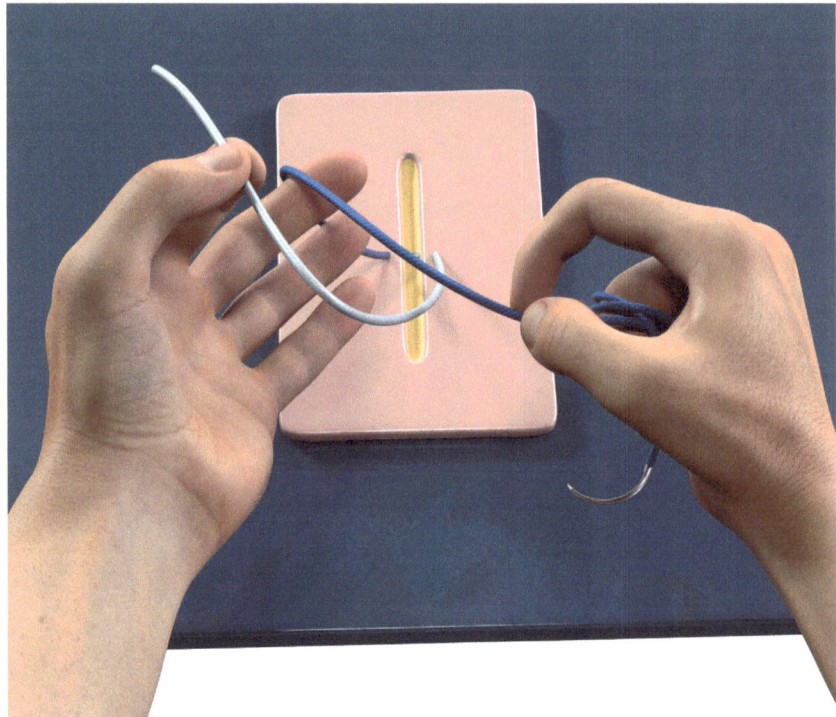

The starting position for a right-handed surgeon is with your right hand facing palm down and your left hand facing up, with the long end of the suture across the palm of your left hand.

Conversely, the starting position for a left-handed surgeon is with your left hand facing palm down and your right hand facing up, with the long end of the suture across the palm of your right hand.

For the left-handed surgeon, subsequent ties will also mirror those used by a right-handed surgeon.

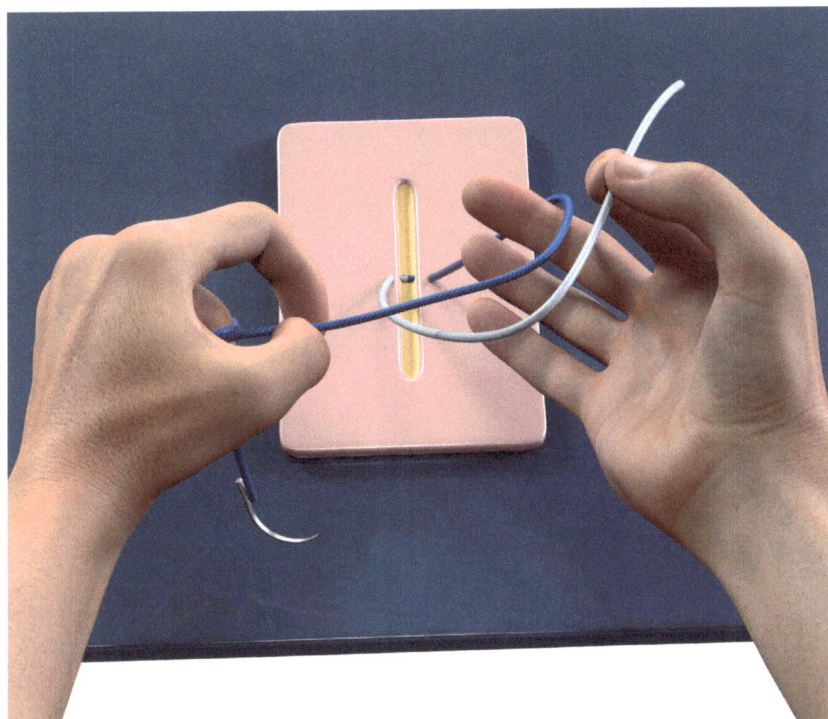

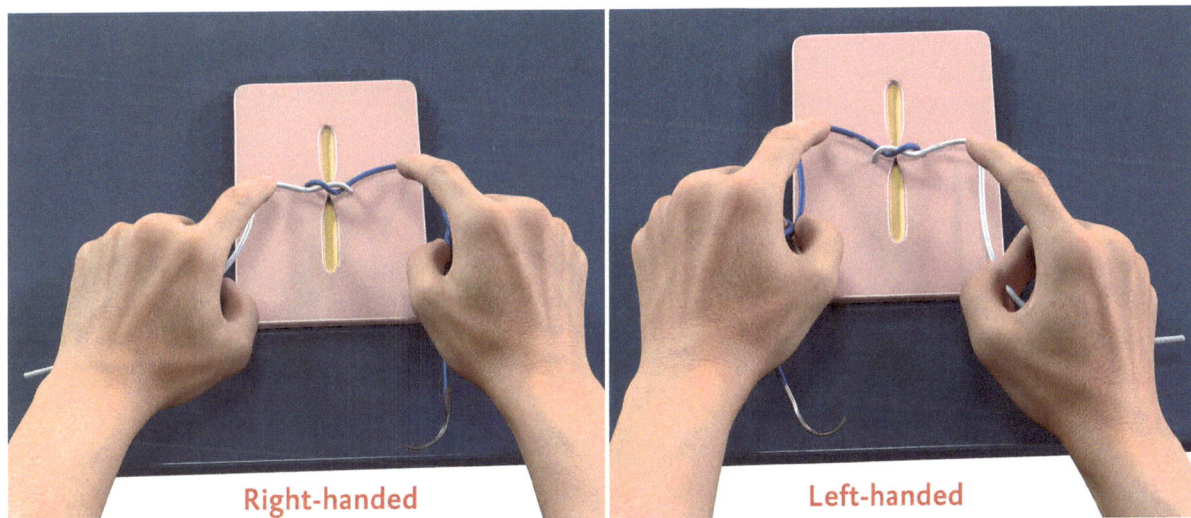

Right-handed   Left-handed

Figure 5.1: Tie down the first throw

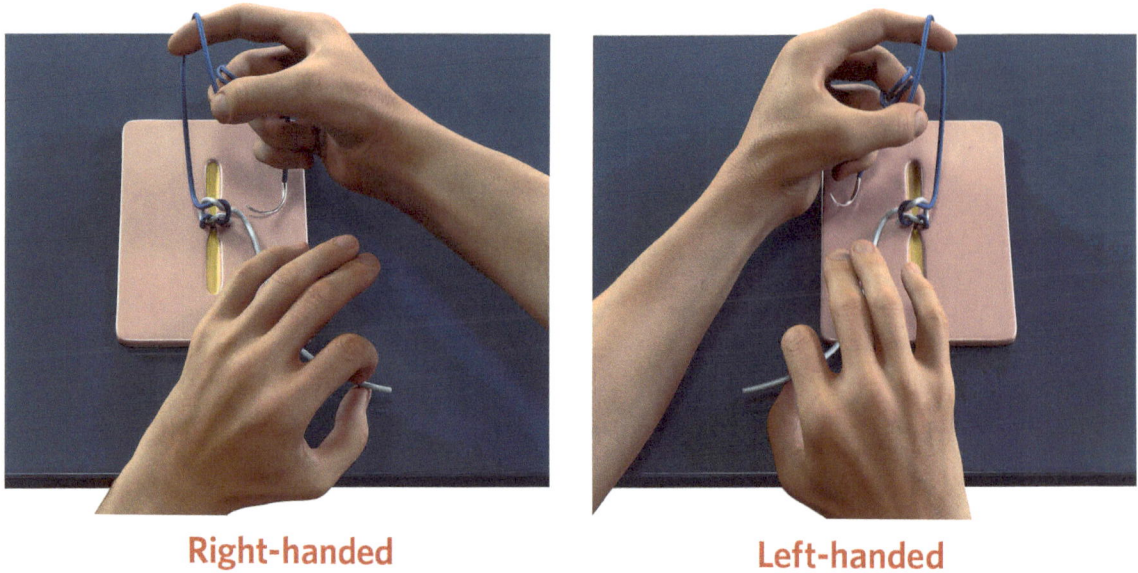

Right-handed   **Left-handed**

Figure 5.2: Tie down the second throw

The most common error I see with junior residents is that they have learned to tie with the wrong hand. That leads to pulling the end of the suture with the needle through the loop. This can lead to injury and is not recommended (except in the rare case of a double-ended suture, where needles are on both sides). Some instructors recommend that surgeons learn to tie one-handed and two-handed ties with both hands, which adds little benefit and creates confusion for the student.

What if the needle is on your dominant side?

Since surgeons generally suture from their dominant towards their non-dominant side, the needle starts on their non-dominant side. Occasionally, surgeons must suture backhanded, or an assistant rather than the surgeon is asked to tie the knot. In those cases, the needle will be on the person's right side tying the knot.

There are three ways of tying a knot in this situation: You can learn to tie with the opposite hand from what you generally use, which I do not recommend. You can pick up the suture as you do when the suture is on the correct side, but you will have to cross your hands to tie the first throw down flat. You can tie the second part of the knot before the first part, and the knot will come down flat. For example, when tying a one-hand tie, do steps 6 - 15; for the second throw, do steps 1-5. For a two-hand tie, do steps 5-9 and then do steps 1-4.

Two-handed Square knot

Step 1: The initial position for tying one-hand and two-hand ties is the same. Hold the short end of the suture with your left hand and the long end further away from you in your right hand. Wrap the suture around the middle part of your right middle finger with your right palm facing down. Curl your right index finger under both the short and long ends of the suture.

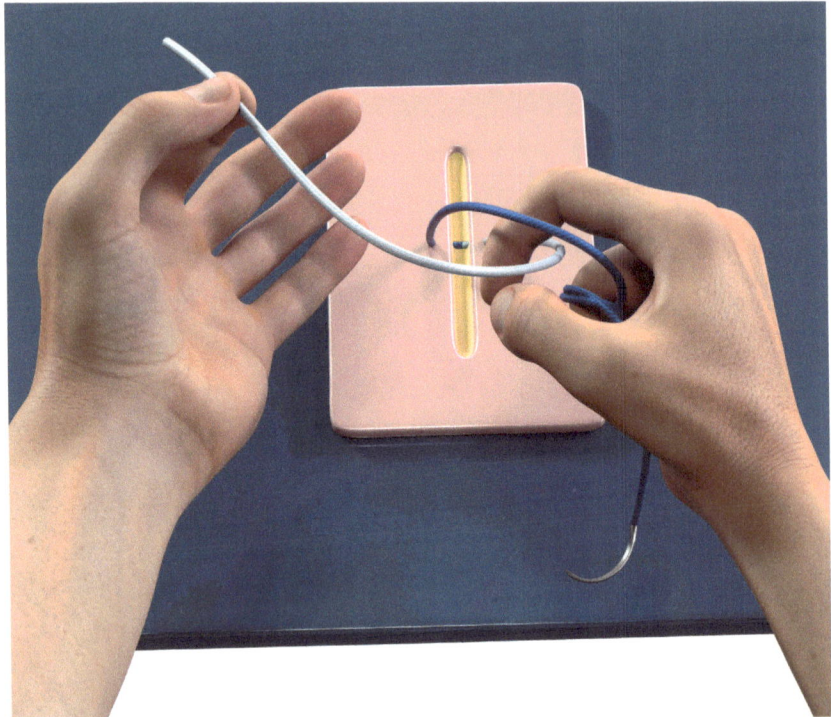

Step 2: Touch your right thumb to your right index finger and put your right thumb under both the short and long ends of the suture. Grasp the short end of the suture between your right thumb and index finger.

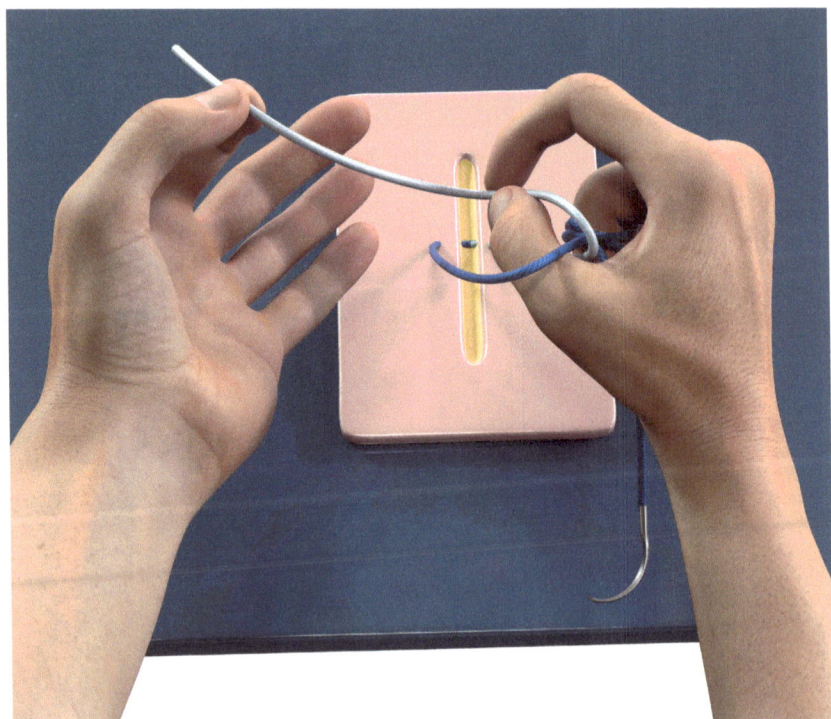

Step 3: Let go of the short end of the suture with your left hand and pull the short end under the long end using your right index finger and thumb. Using your left thumb and middle finger, grasp the short end of the suture.

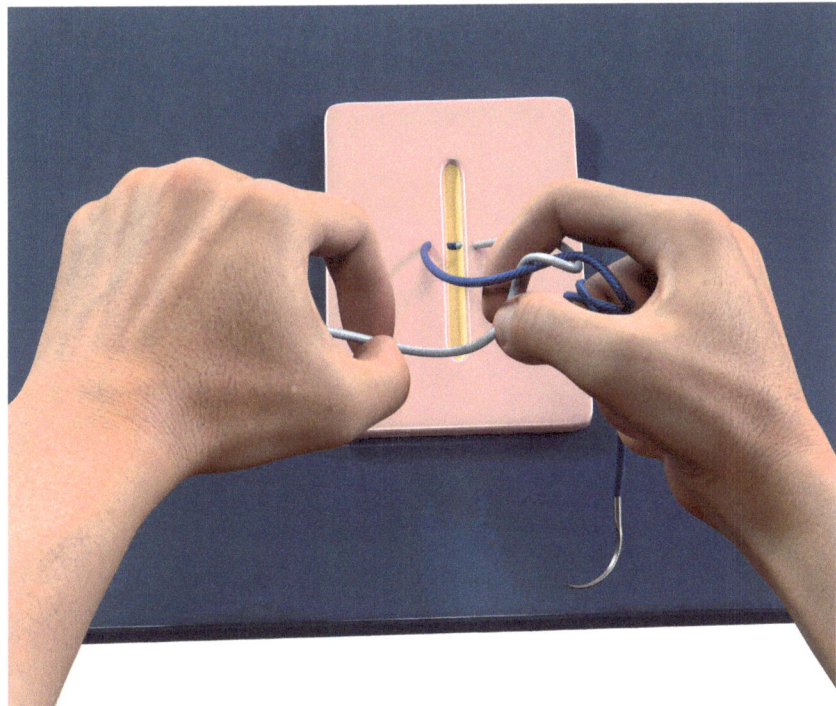

Step 4: Use your two index fingers to pull the suture down flat.

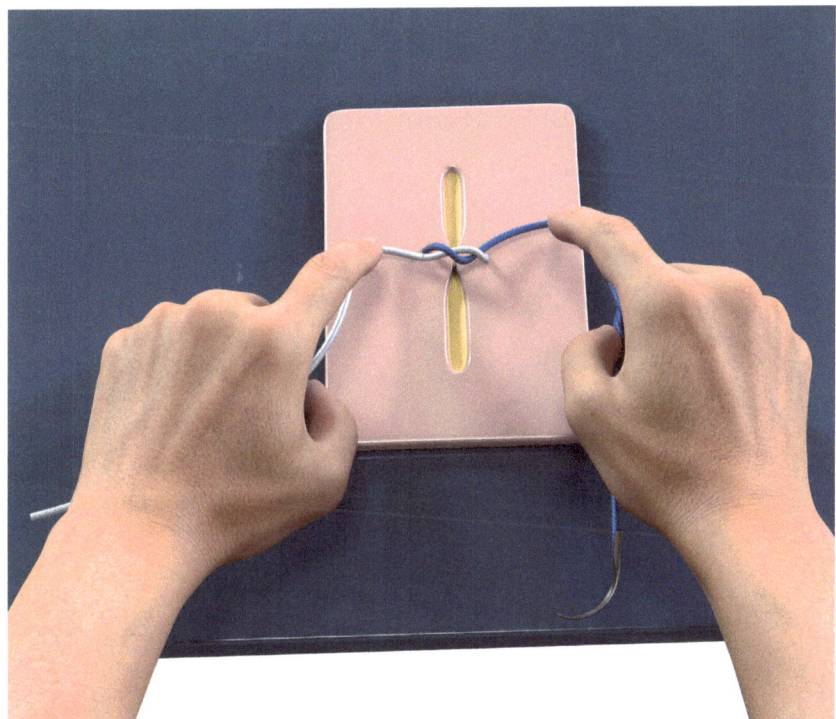

Step 5: Hook your right thumb under the long end of the suture.

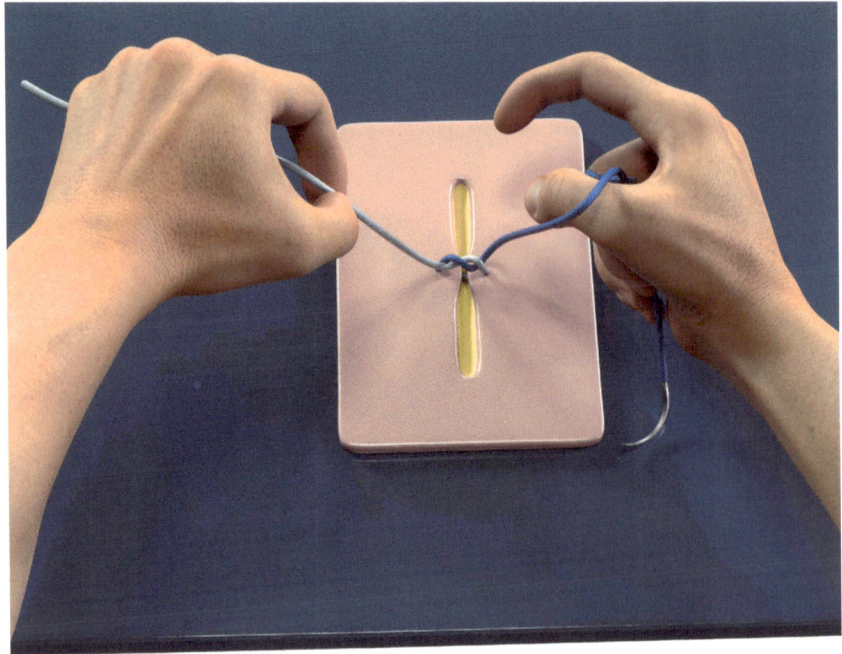

Step 6: Using your left hand, pull the short end of the suture over your right thumb to form a loop.

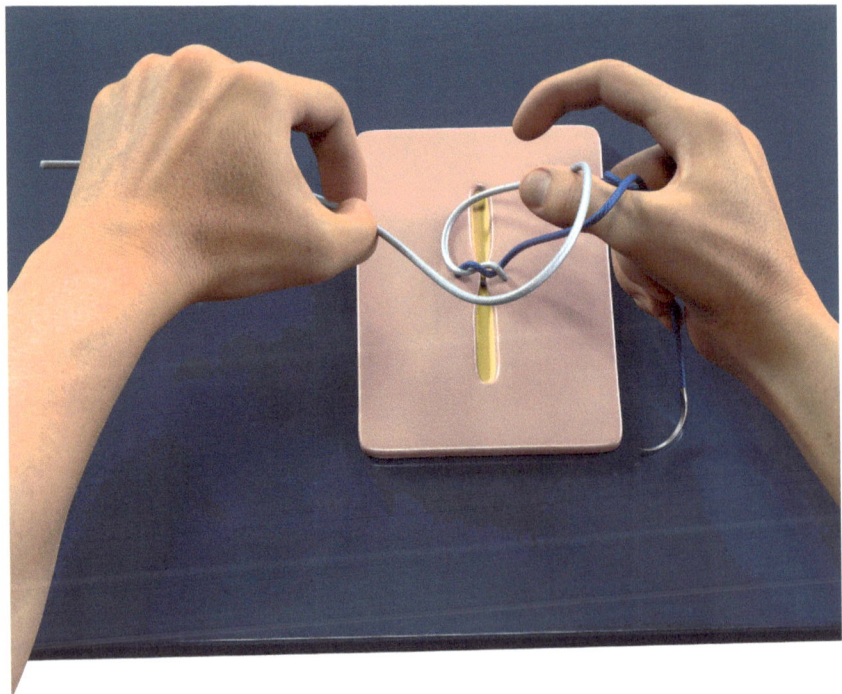

Step 7: Bend your right index finger to touch your right thumb and bring your index finger under the loop. Grab the short end of the suture between your right thumb and index finger.

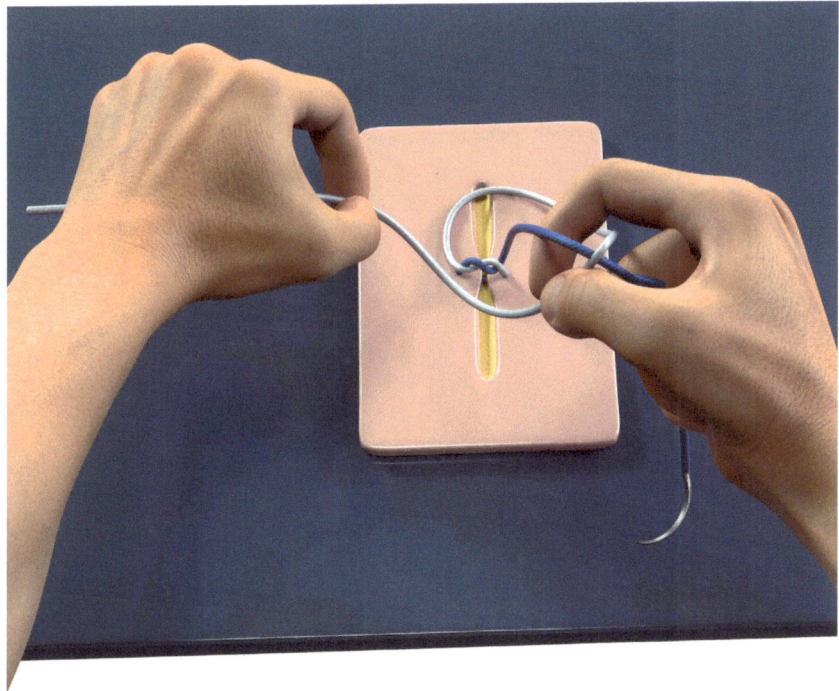

Step 8: Let go of the short end of the suture held by your left hand. Bring your right thumb back under the loop, bringing the short end of the suture with it. Re-grab the short end with your left hand.

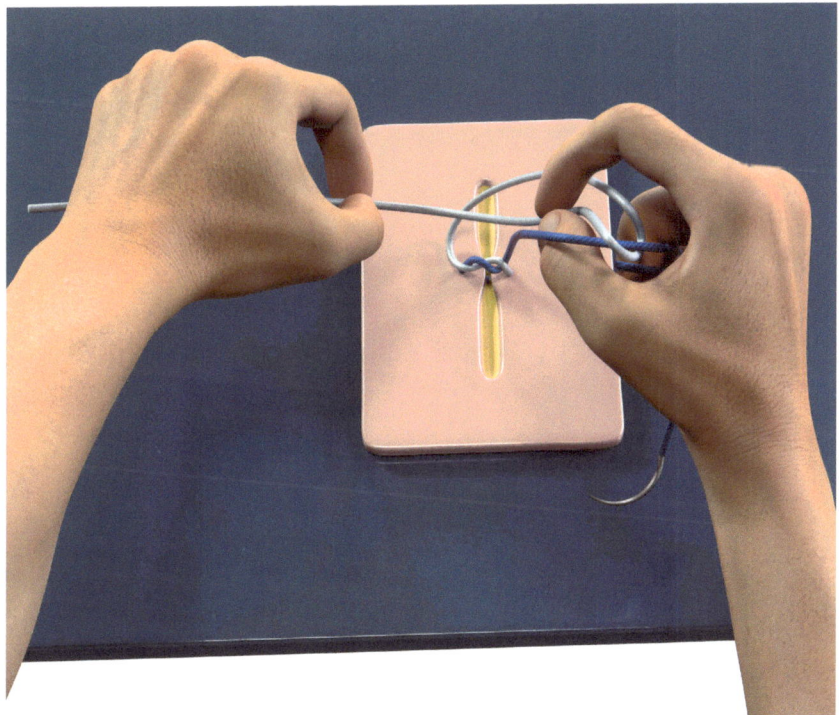

Step 9: Pull the knot down by pulling the short end toward you and the long end away from you (90 degrees to your first knot).

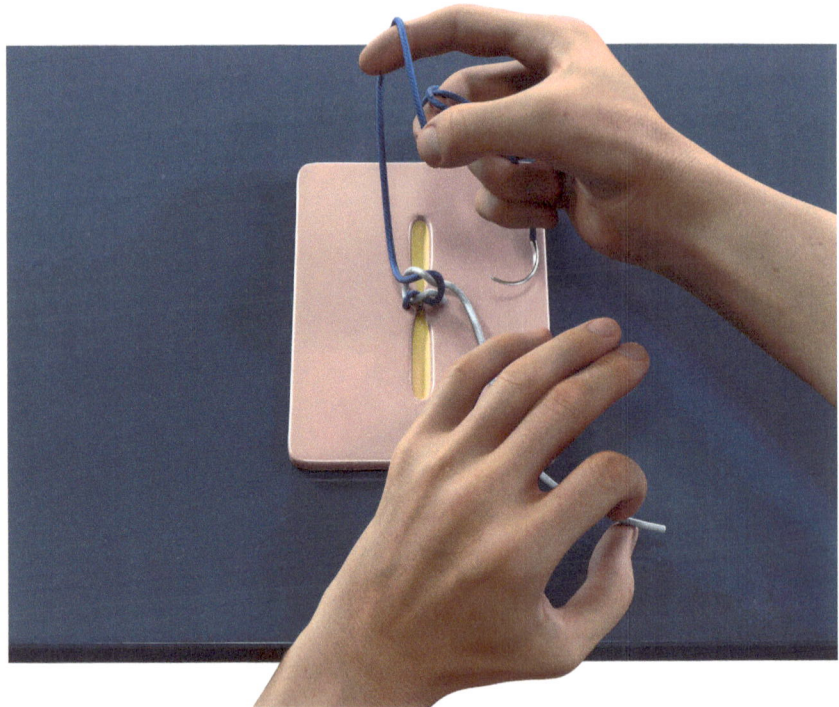

Step 10: Tie subsequent throws away from and towards you, repeating steps 2-8.

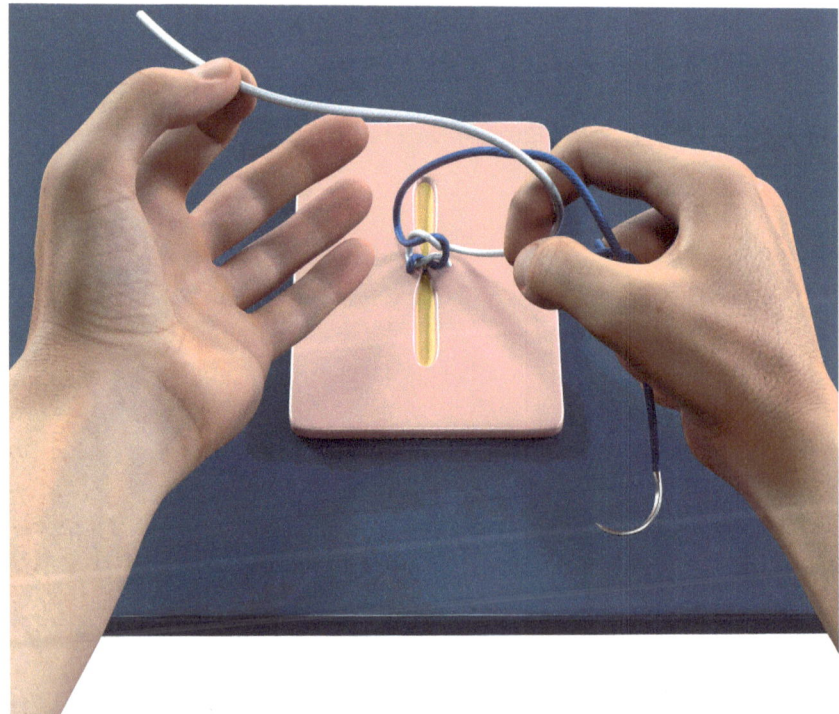

Video of two-handed tie:
https://vimeo.com/190934988

Hand tying a Surgeon's knot

Double wrap two-handed method

This technique is similar to tying a two-hand square knot, but an extra wrap is added to the first throw.

Step 1: The initial position for tying one-hand and two-hand ties is the same. Hold the short end of the suture with your left hand and the long end further away from you in your right hand. Wrap the suture around the middle part of your right middle finger with your right palm facing down. Curl your right index finger under both the short and long ends of the suture.

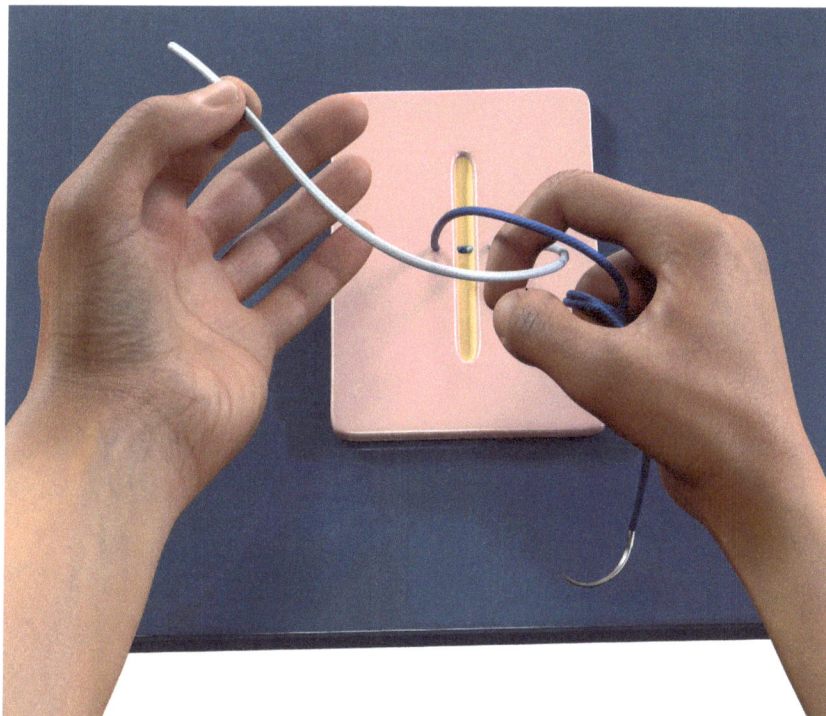

Step 2: Touch your right thumb to your right index finger and put your right thumb under both the short and long ends of the suture. Grasp the short end of the suture between your right thumb and index finger.

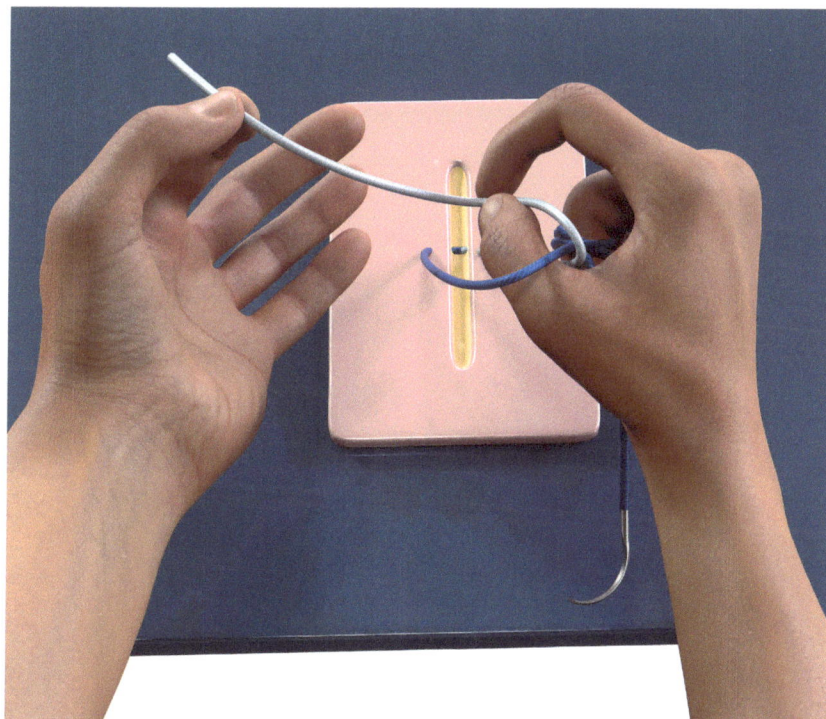

Step 3: Let go of the short end of the suture with your left hand and pull it under the long end using your right index finger and thumb. Grasp the short end of the suture with your left hand.

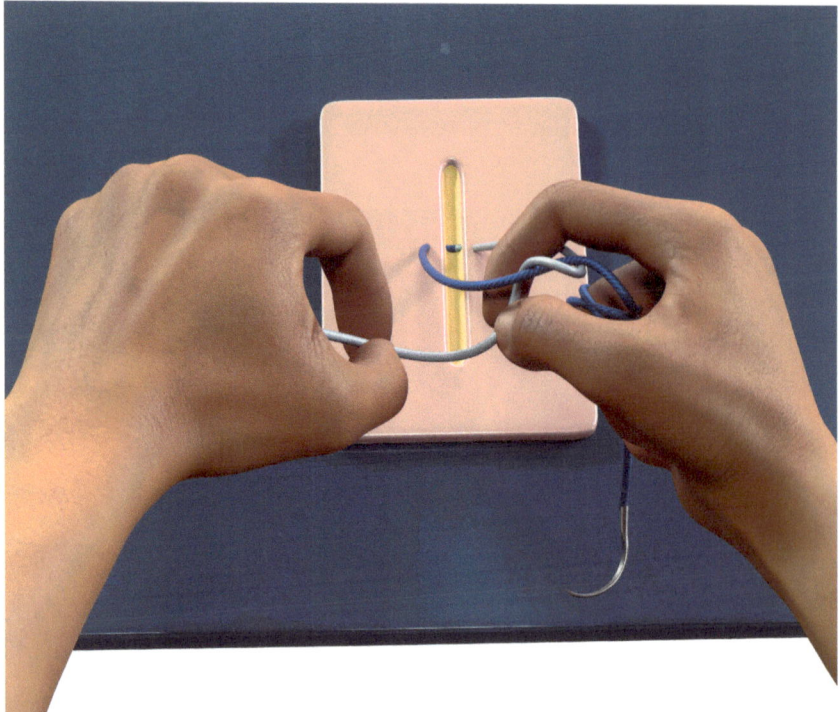

Step 4: Place your right thumb under the loop and use your left hand to move the suture away from you so that it can be grasped between your right thumb and index finger.

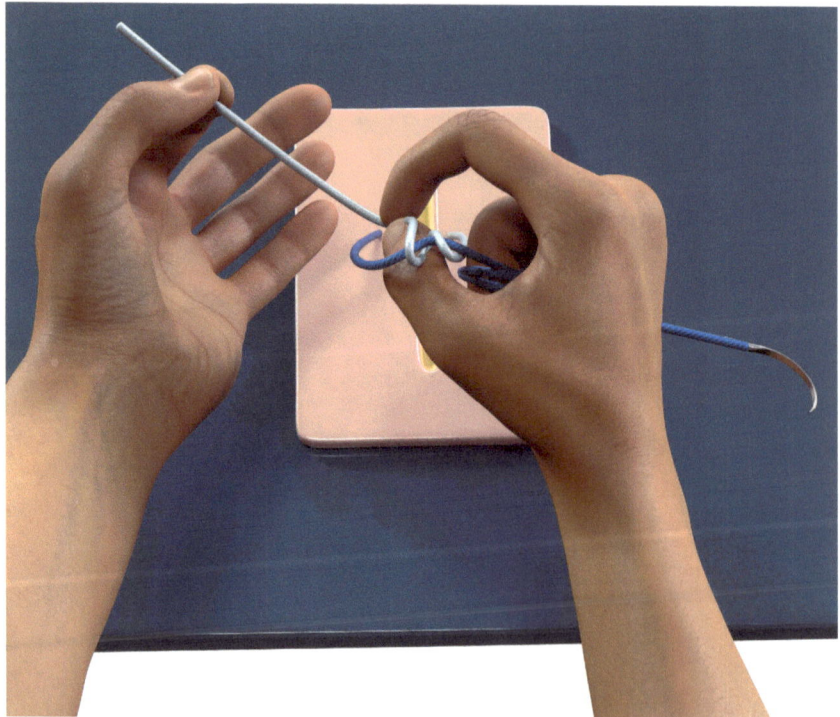

Step 5: Let go of the short end of the suture with your left hand and pull it under the long end using your right index finger and thumb. Re-grasp the short end of the suture with your left hand.

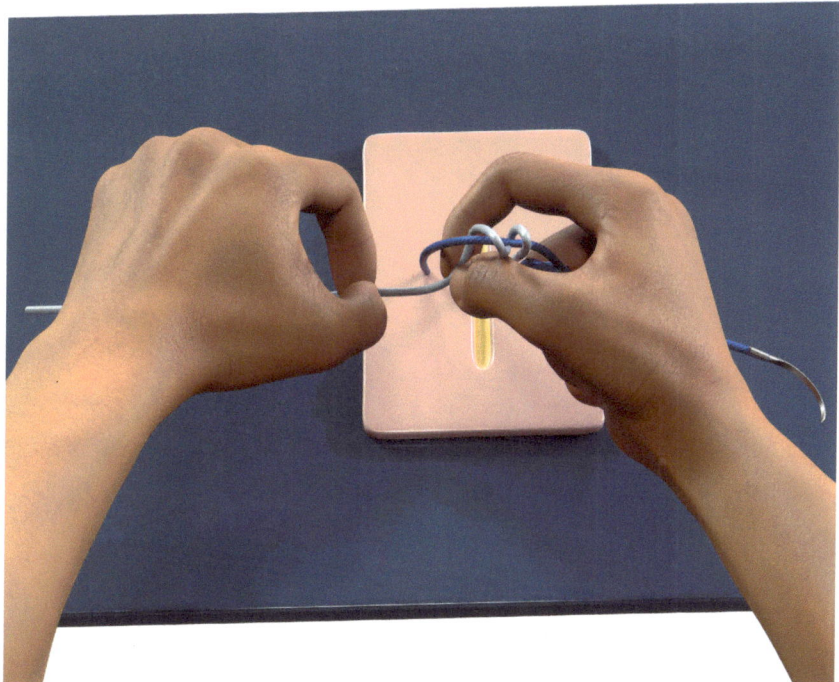

Step 6: Use the index fingers of both hands to tighten the first throw down.

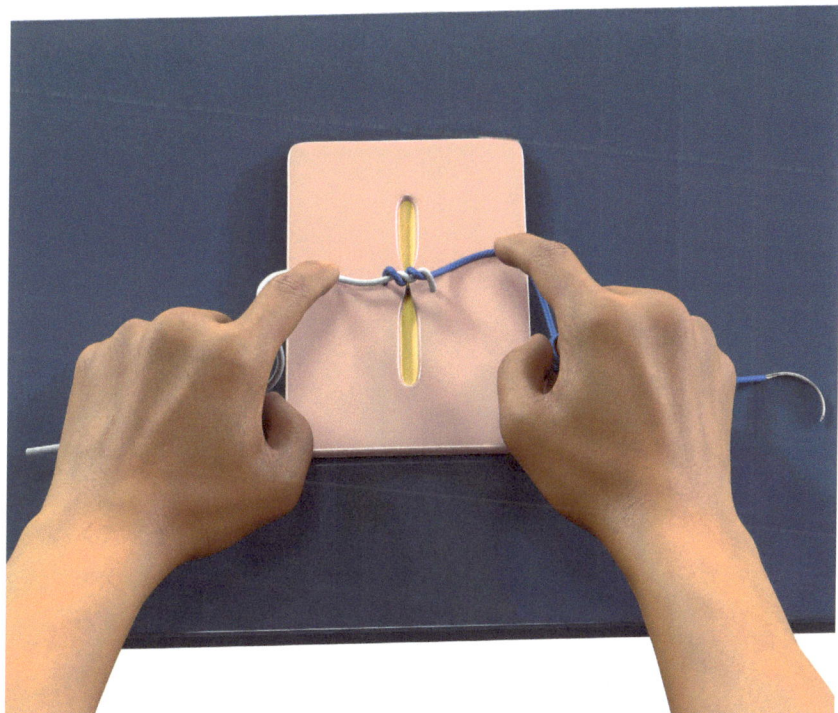

Step 7: Hook your right thumb under the long end of the suture.

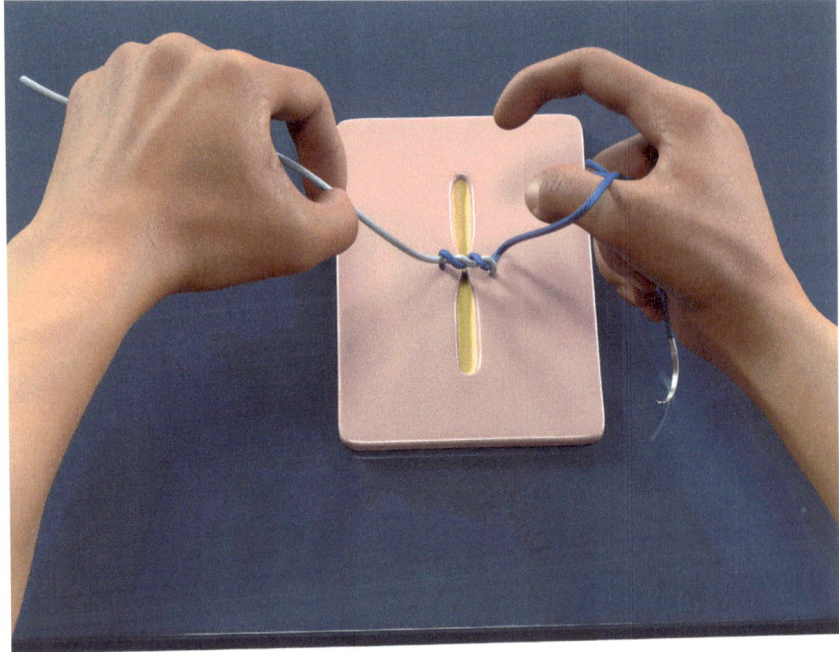

Step 8: Using your left hand, pull the short end of the suture over your right thumb to form a loop.

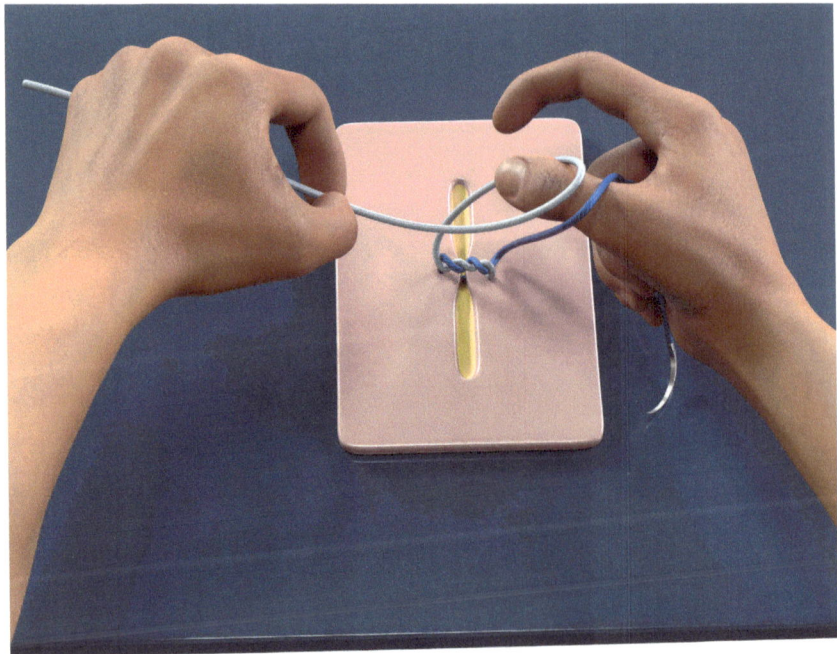

Step 9: Bend your right index finger to touch your right thumb and bring your index finger under the loop. Grasp the short end of the suture between your right thumb and index finger.

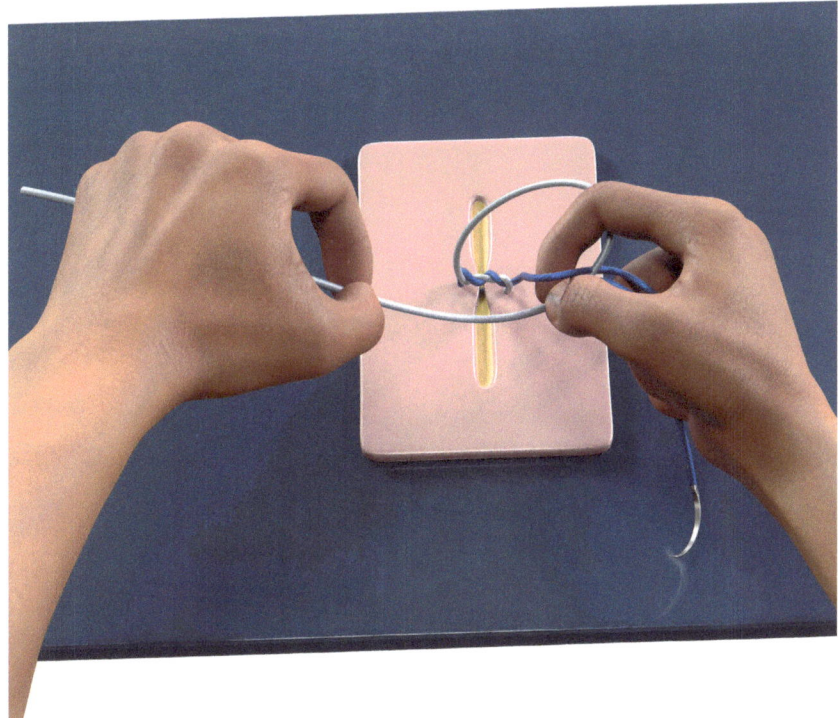

Step 10: Let go of the short end of the suture with your left hand. Bring the short end under the loop with your right thumb. Re-grasp the short end with your left hand.

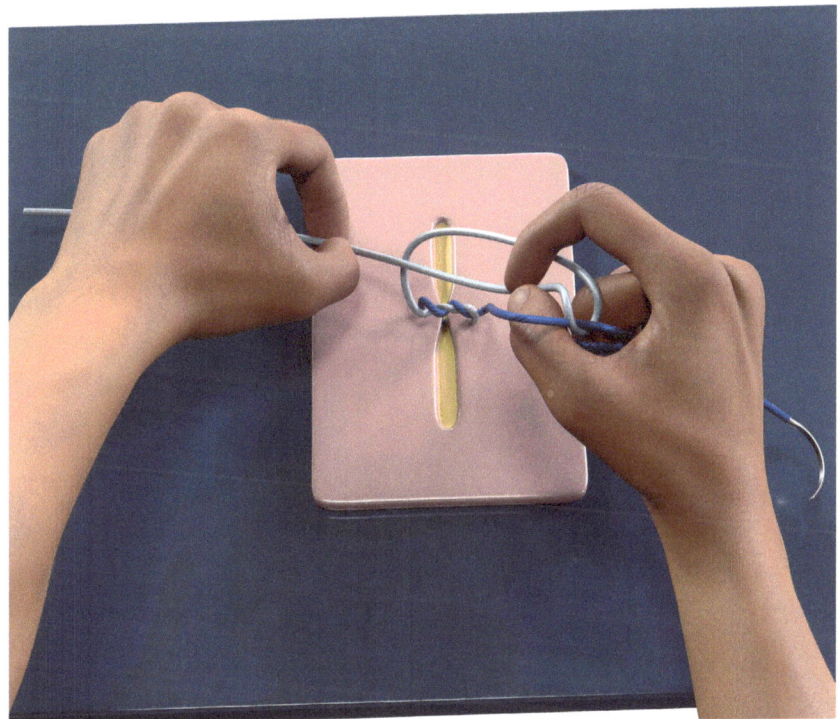

Step 11: Pull the knot down by pulling the short end toward you and the long end away from you (90 degrees to your first knot).

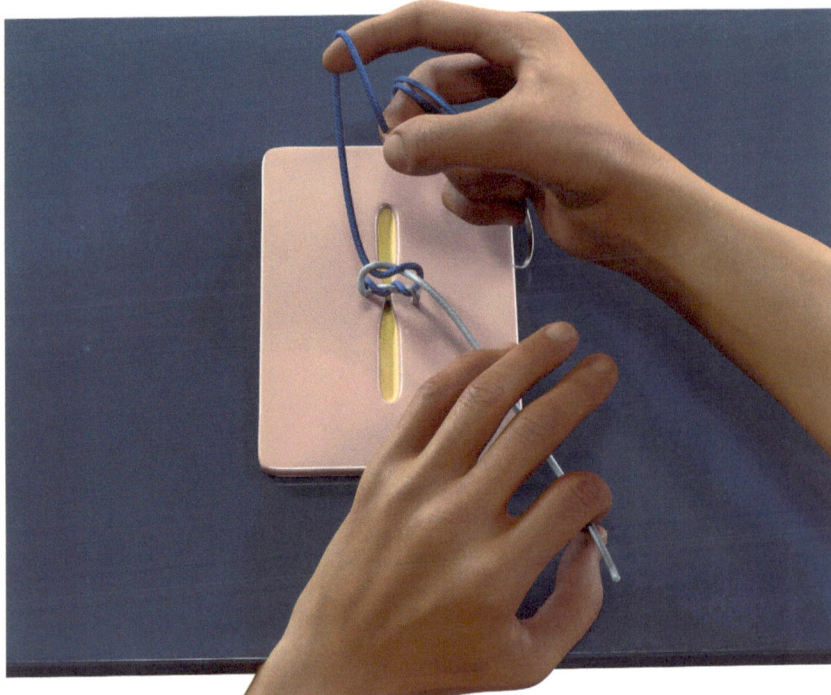

Double wrap one-handed and one-hand, two-hand method

This technique is similar to that used to tie a one-hand Square knot, but an extra wrap is added using a one-hand or two-hand technique for the second wrap.

Step 1: Using your right hand and keeping your left palm up, bring the long end of the suture across the palm of your left hand. Hold the suture away from your other fingers between your left thumb and index finger.

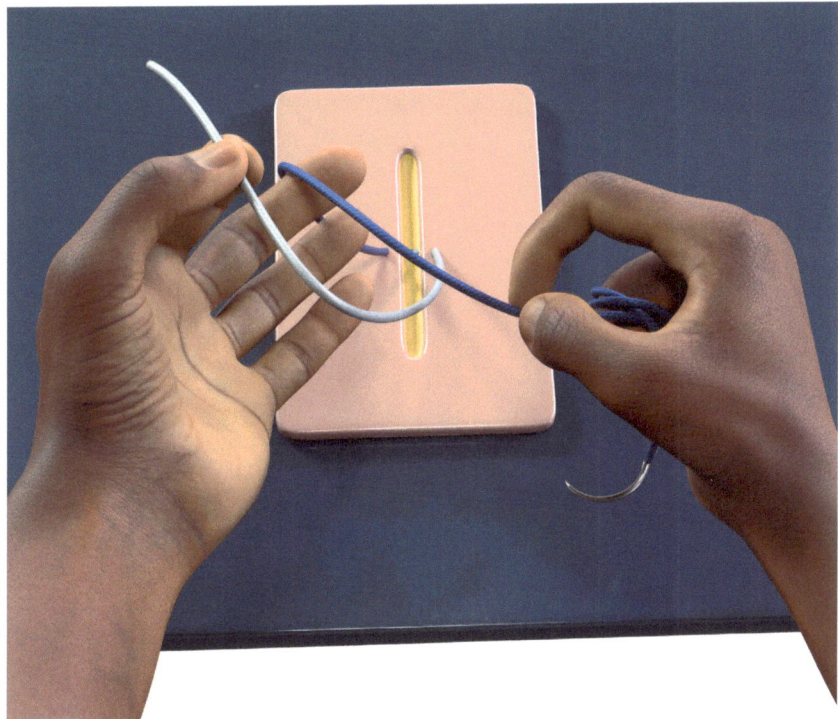

Step 2: Bend your left middle finger under the short end of the suture, preparing to catch the short end between the back of your left middle finger and front of your left ring finger.

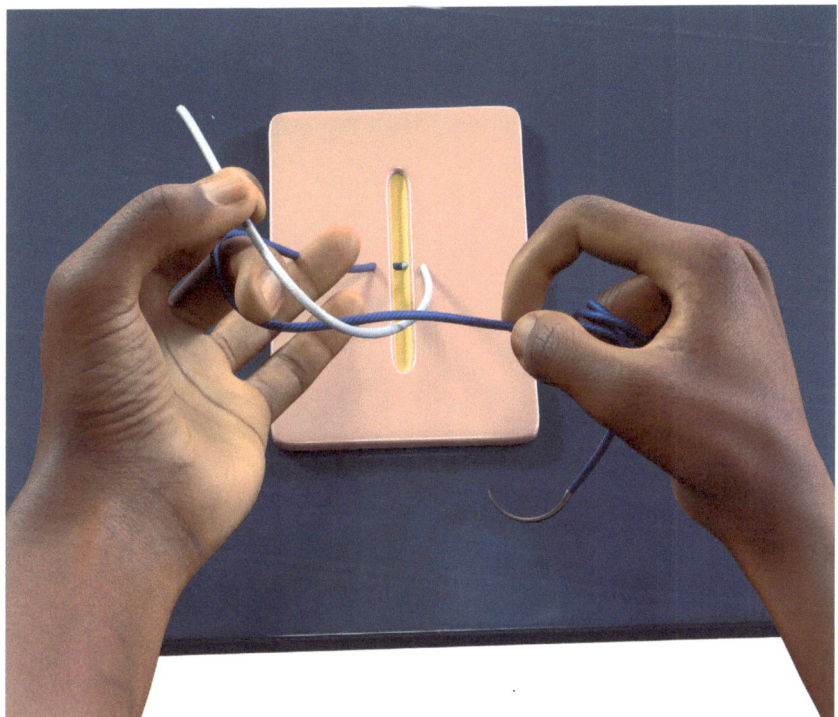

Step 3: Catch the short end of the suture between your left middle and ring fingers and release the grip on the suture between your thumb and index finger.

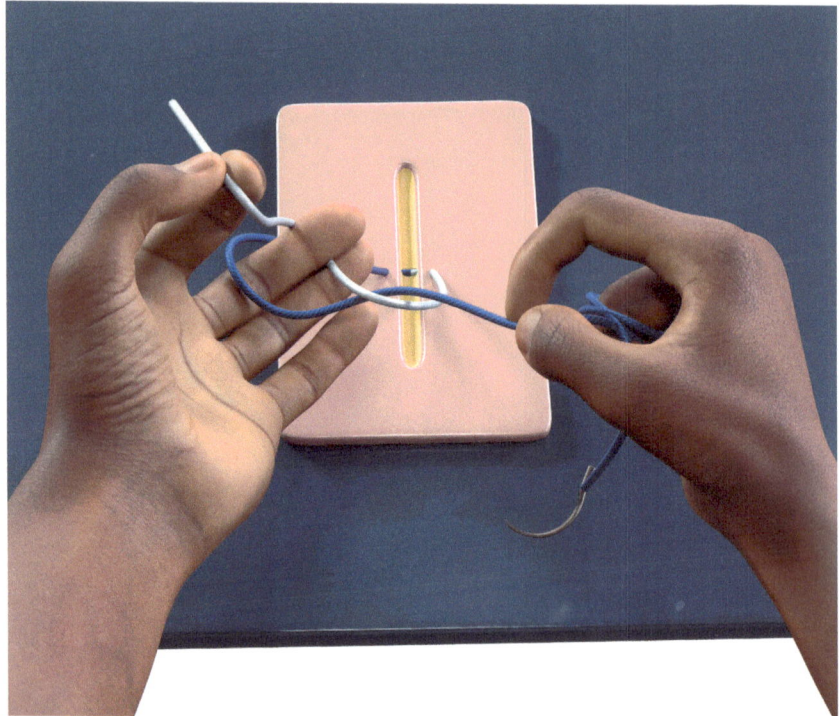

Step 4: Pull the tip of the suture's short end under the suture's long end.

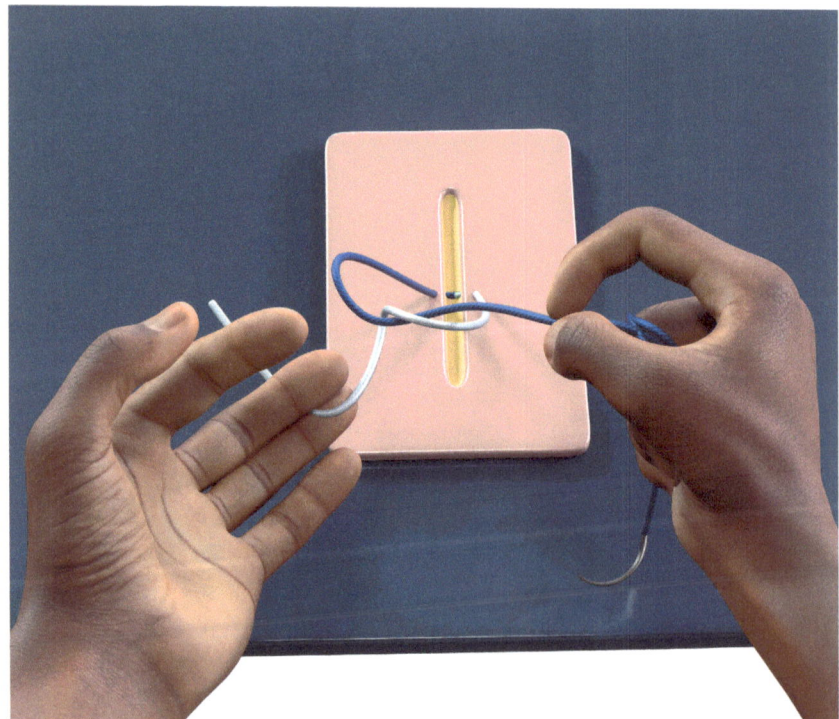

Step 5: Place your left hand back under the loop formed by the suture, keeping your palm face up. Grasp the short end of the suture between your right middle and ring fingers.

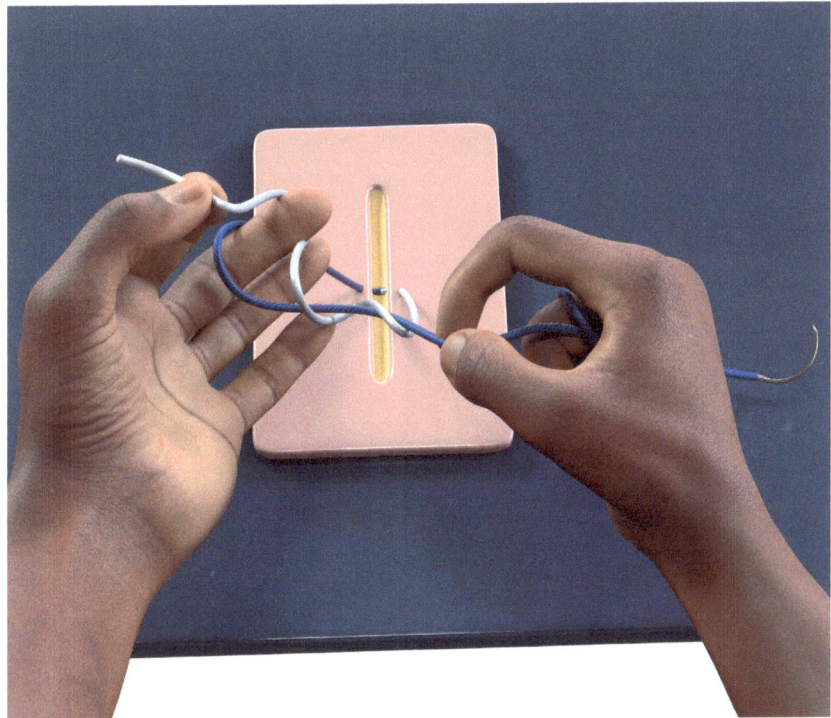

Alternatively, you can tie the second throw with your right hand, using the same method as a two-handed Surgeon's knot.

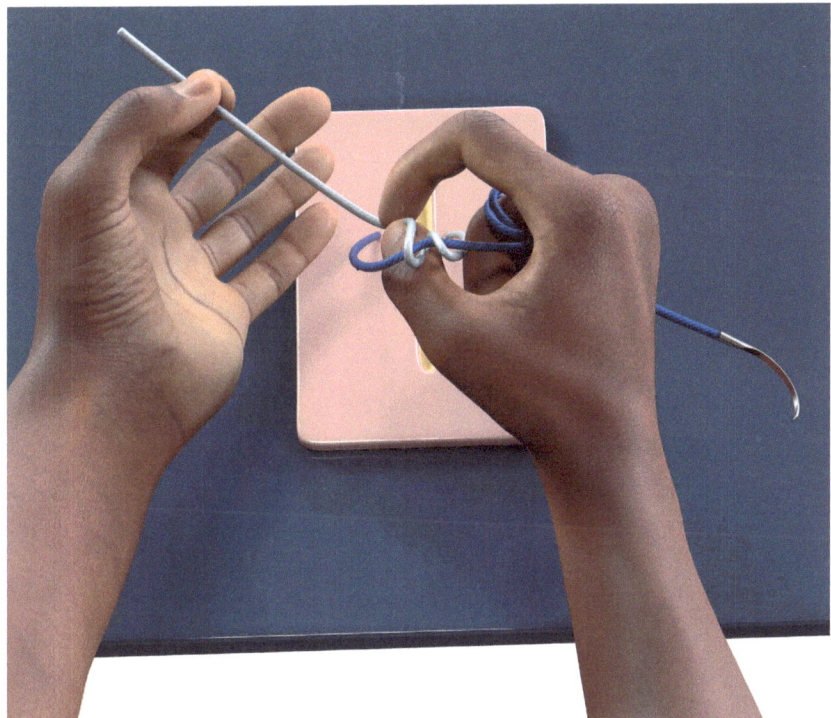

Step 6: Pull the suture back through the loop and tighten the knot with your index fingers. Form the second throw either by following steps 5 - 9 for a two-handed Square knot, or steps 6 - 15 for a one-handed Square knot.

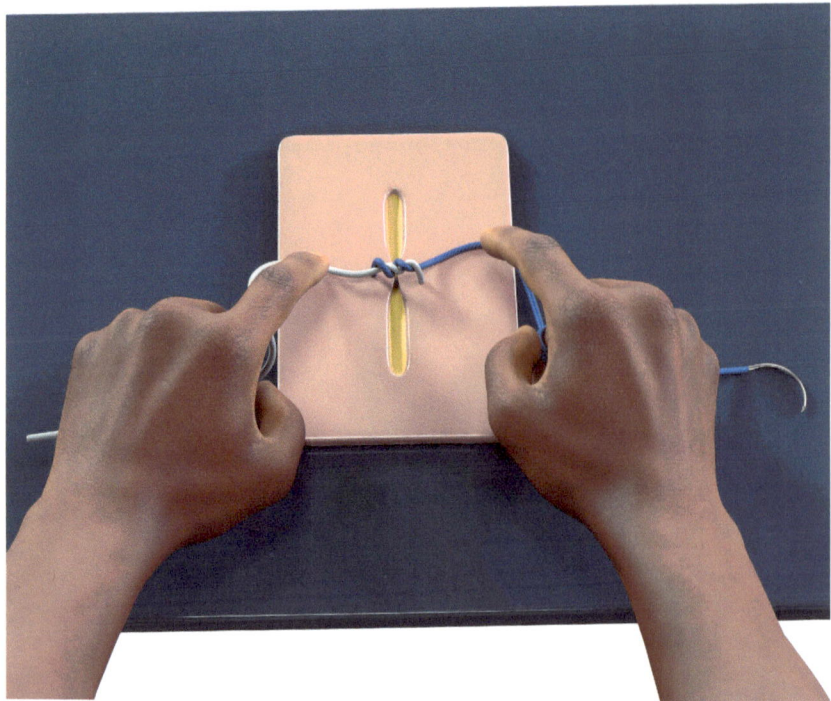

Double one-hand wrap method

This technique is similar to that used to tie a one-handed Square knot, but a one-handed throw with the opposite hand adds a simultaneous extra wrap to the first loop. It is faster than the previous techniques but has the disadvantage of pulling the needle through the loop, potentially causing an injury.

Step 1: Using your right hand and keeping your left palm up, bring the long end of the suture across the palm of your left hand. Grasp the end of the suture between your left middle and ring fingers. Curve your right index finger around the needle end of the suture.

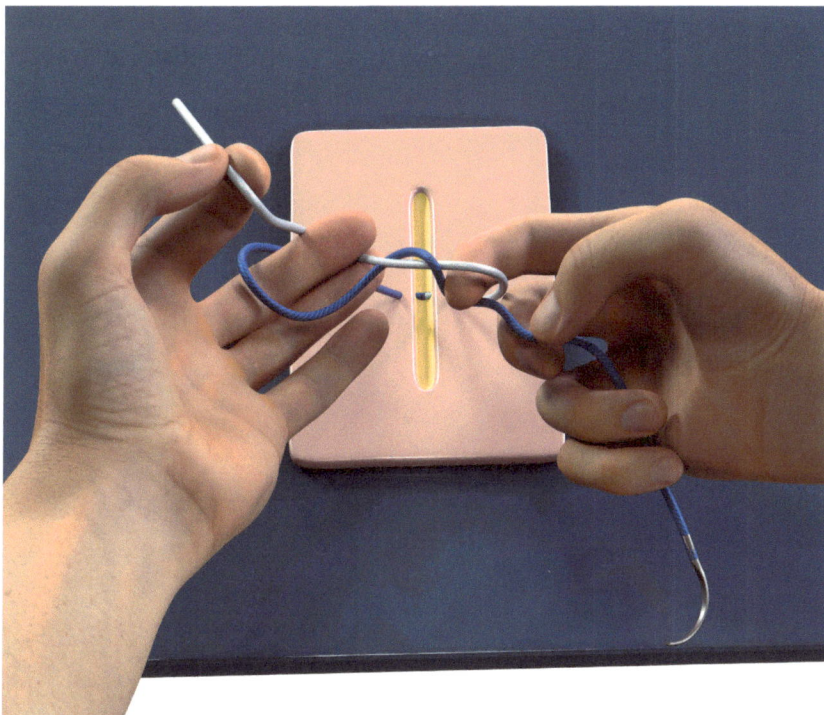

Step 2: Holding the short end of the suture with your left middle and ring fingers, pull it through the loop. Simultaneously pull the other end of the suture through the loop with your right index finger. Grasp the suture with your right hand and pull the needle through the loop. Pull the knot down using both index fingers.

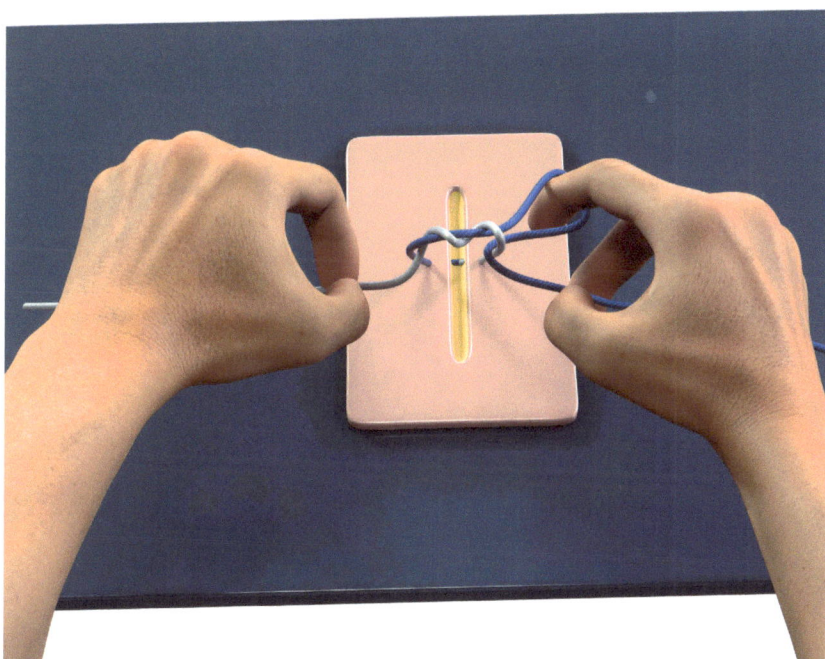

Tying a Nicky knot

One-handed method

A Nicky knot can start a running suture. It is also helpful when tissue is under tension, and you want to appose tissue reliably without back slipping. It has less chance of back slipping during tying than a Granny or Square noose but is not secure. To secure it, you must add flat Square knots after finishing the Nicky knot.

The first throw of a Nicky knot is the same as tying a Surgeon's knot, but the second throw is done as a Granny knot.

Step 1: Using your right hand and keeping your left palm up, bring the long end of the suture across the palm of your left hand.

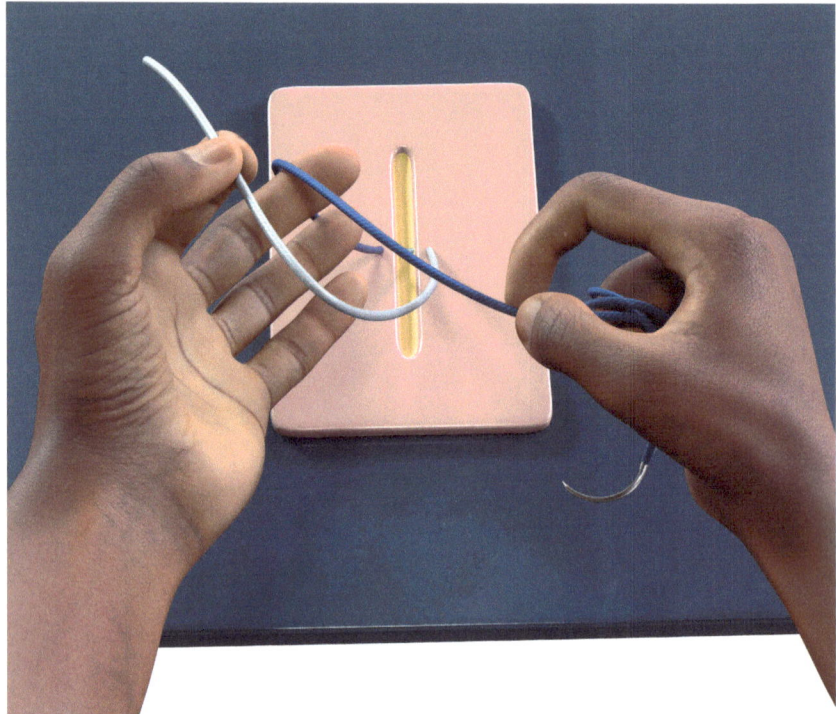

Step 2: Bend your left middle finger under the short end of the suture, preparing to catch the short end between the back of your left middle finger and the front of your left ring finger.

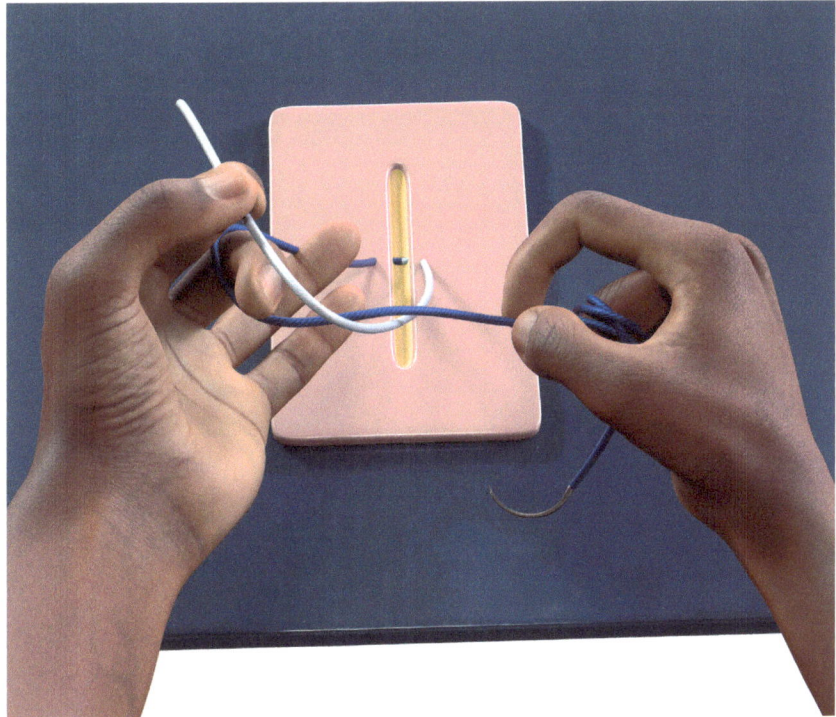

Step 3: Catch the short end of the suture between your left middle and ring fingers. Release the grip on the suture between your thumb and index finger.

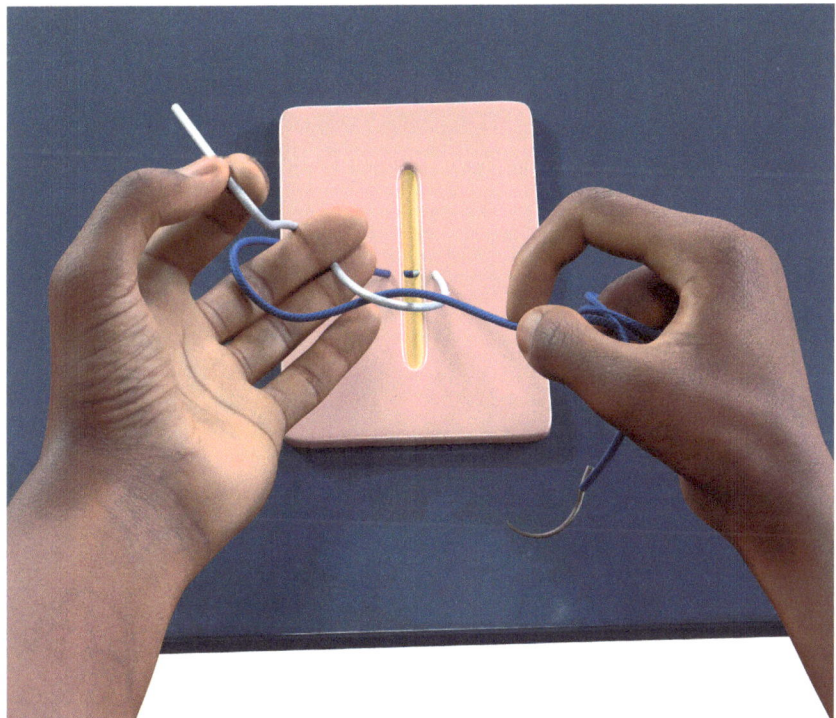

Step 4: Pull the tip of the suture's short end under the suture's long end.

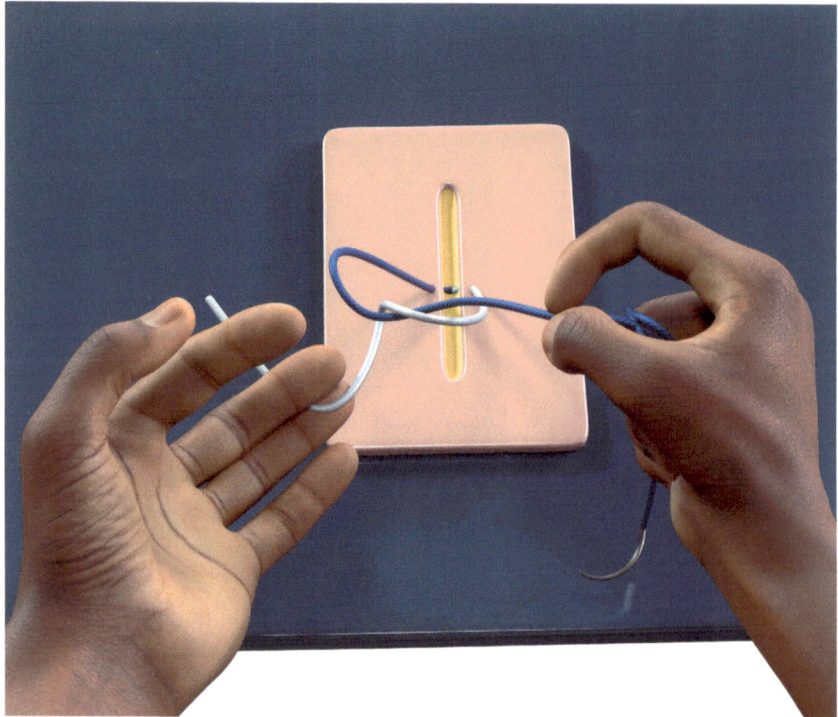

Step 5: Place your left hand back under the loop formed by the suture, keeping your palm face up. Grasp the short end of the suture between your right middle and ring fingers.

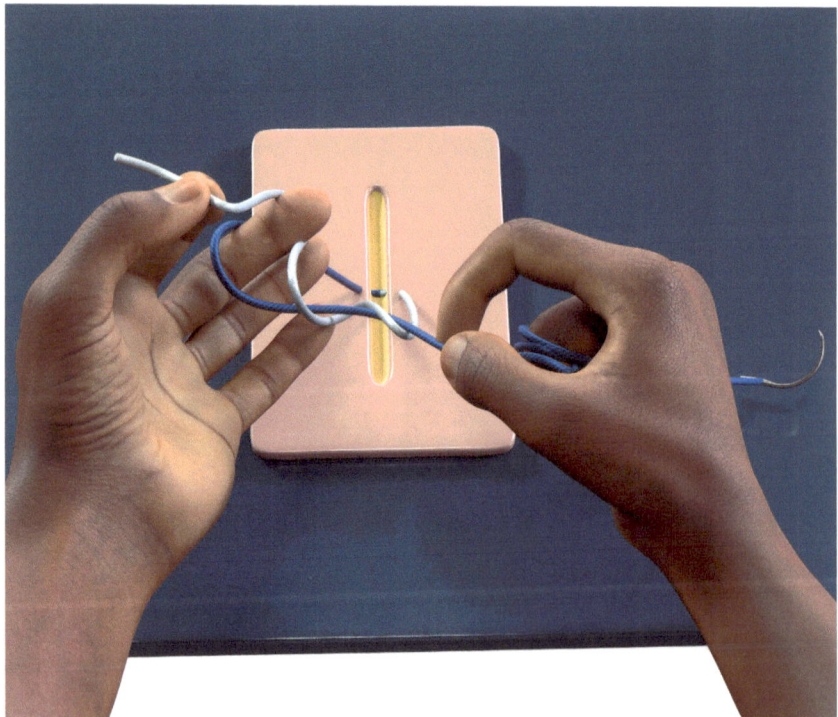

Step 6: Pull up on the suture with your right hand to form a noose. Pull up with your left hand to tighten the short end around the long end, dressing the knot.

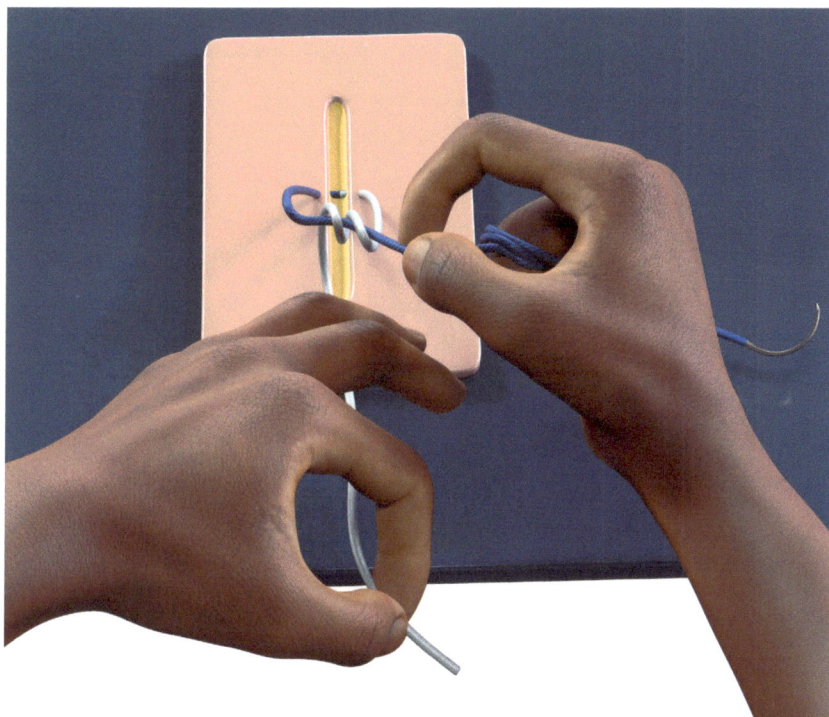

Step 7: Turn your left palm up. Using your right hand, bring the long end of the suture across the palm of your left hand.

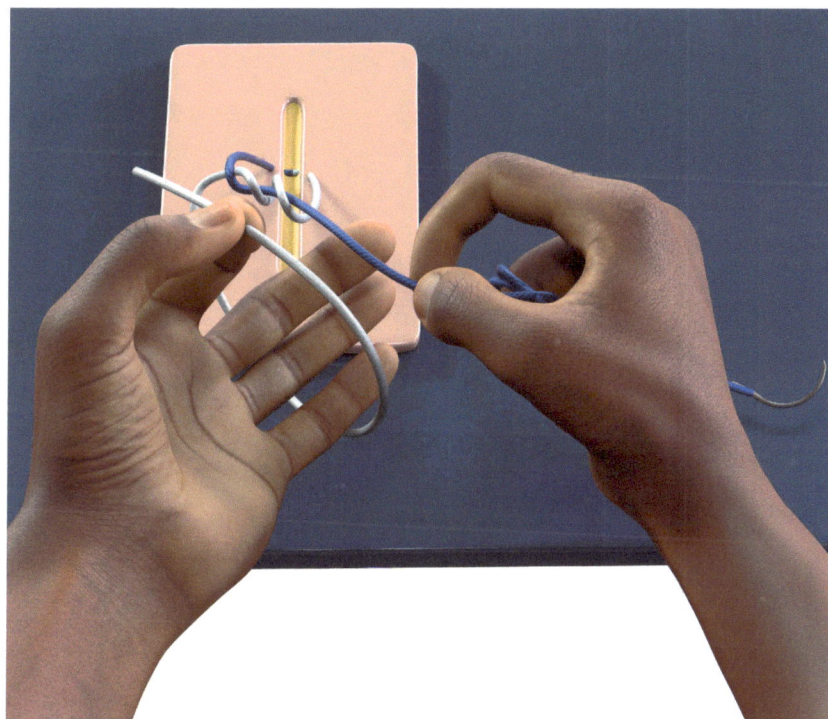

Step 8: Bend your left middle finger under the short end of the suture. Prepare to catch the short end of the suture between the back of your left middle finger and the front of your left ring finger.

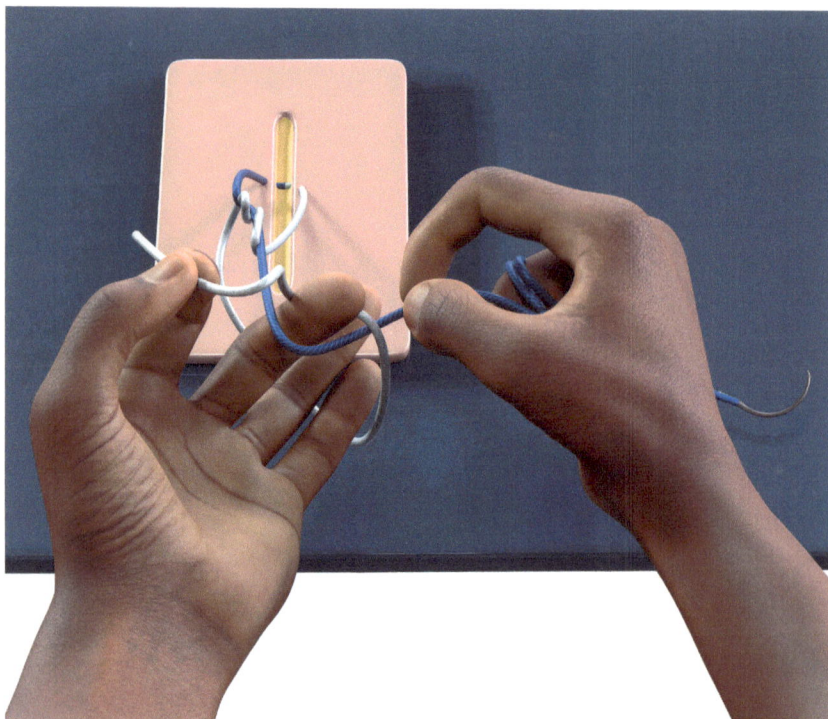

Step 9: Grasp the short end of the suture between your left middle and ring fingers. Release the grip on the suture between your thumb and index finger. Pull the tip of the short end of the suture under the long end.

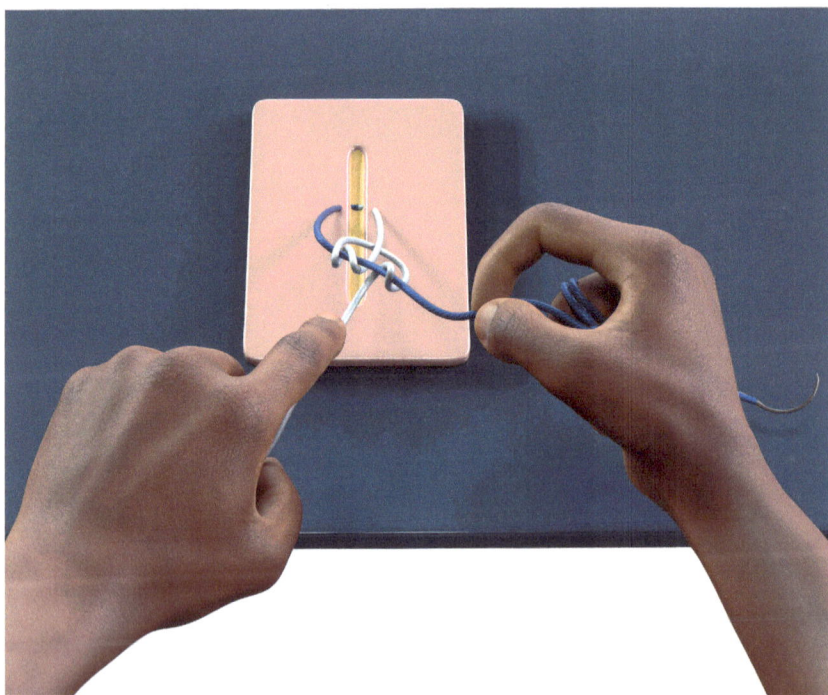

Step 10: Pull up on the suture with your right hand to form a noose. Pull up with your left hand to tighten the short end around the long end, dressing the knot. Using your left index finger, slide the knot down to tighten.

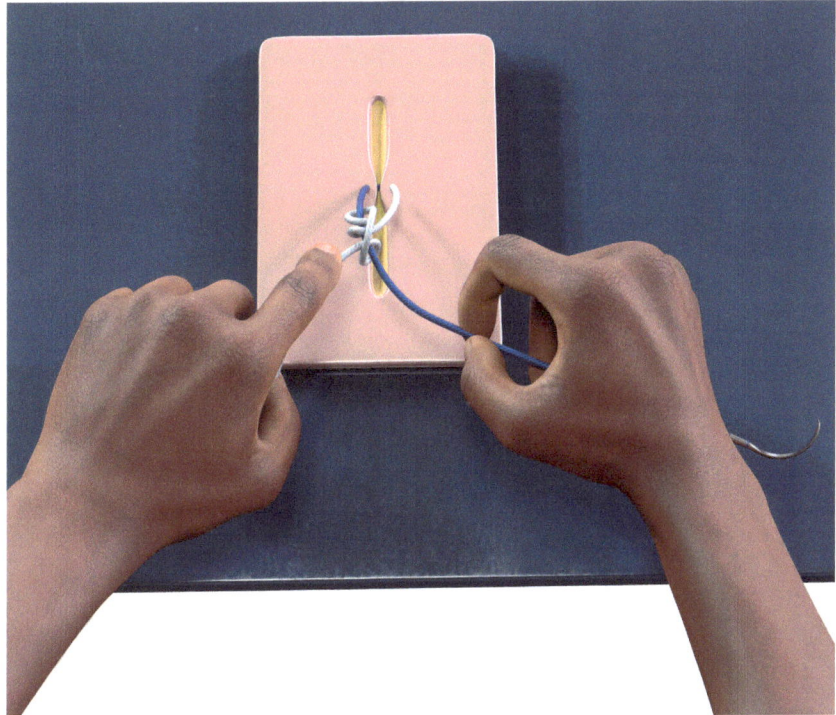

Tying a Revo knot

A Revo knot can be tied with a series of one or two-hand throws. The technique described below starts by tying a Granny knot with one-handed throws.

Step 1: Using your right hand and keeping your left palm up, bring the long end of the suture across the palm of your left hand.

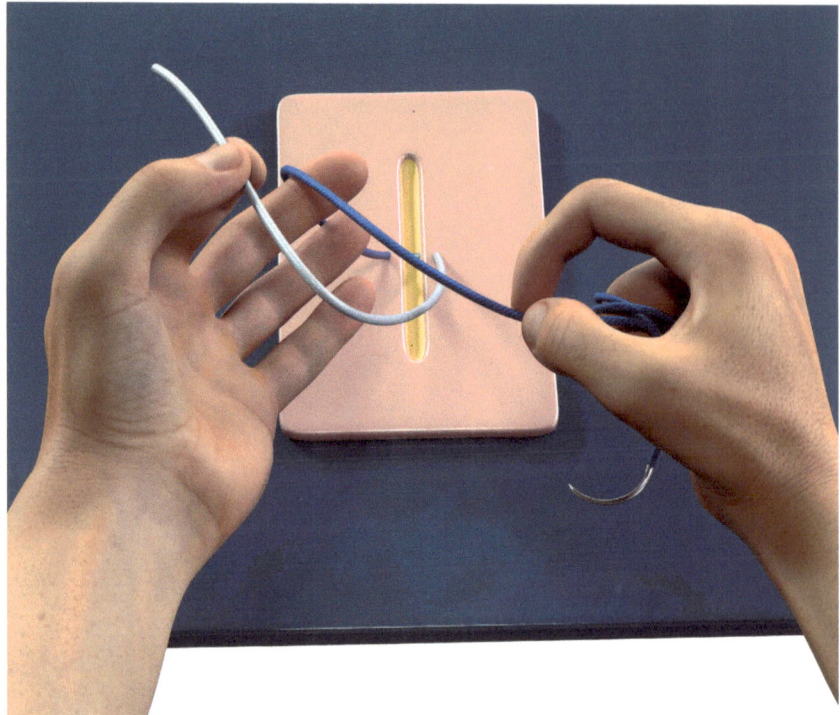

Step 2: Bend your left middle finger under the short end of the suture, preparing to catch the short end of the suture between the back of your left middle finger and front of your left ring finger.

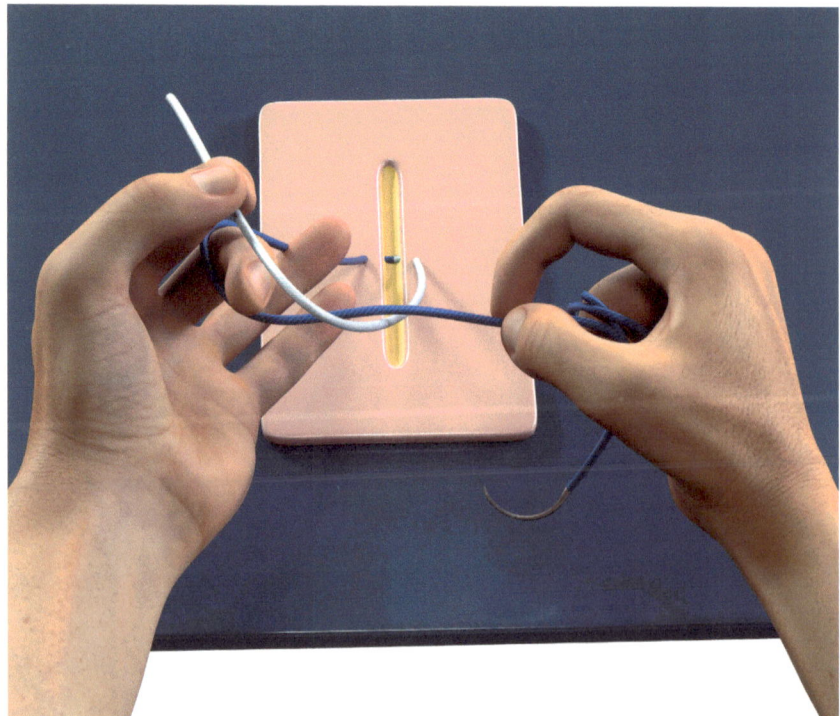

Step 3: Catch the short end of the suture between your left middle and ring finger and release the grip on the suture between your thumb and index finger.

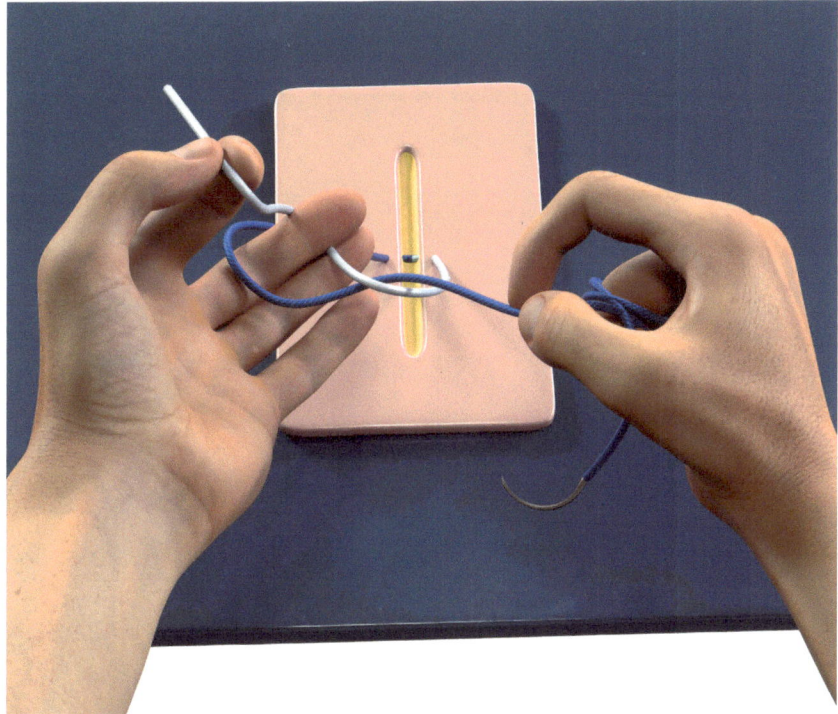

Step 4: Pull the tip of the suture's short end under the suture's long end.

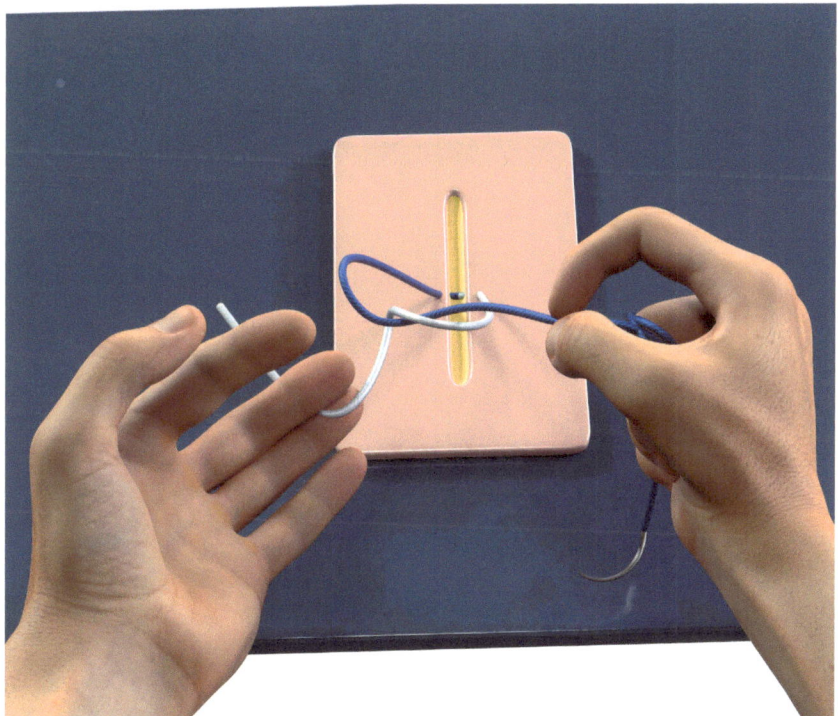

Step 5: Pull up on the long end of the suture to convert the overhand knot to a noose and push the knot down.

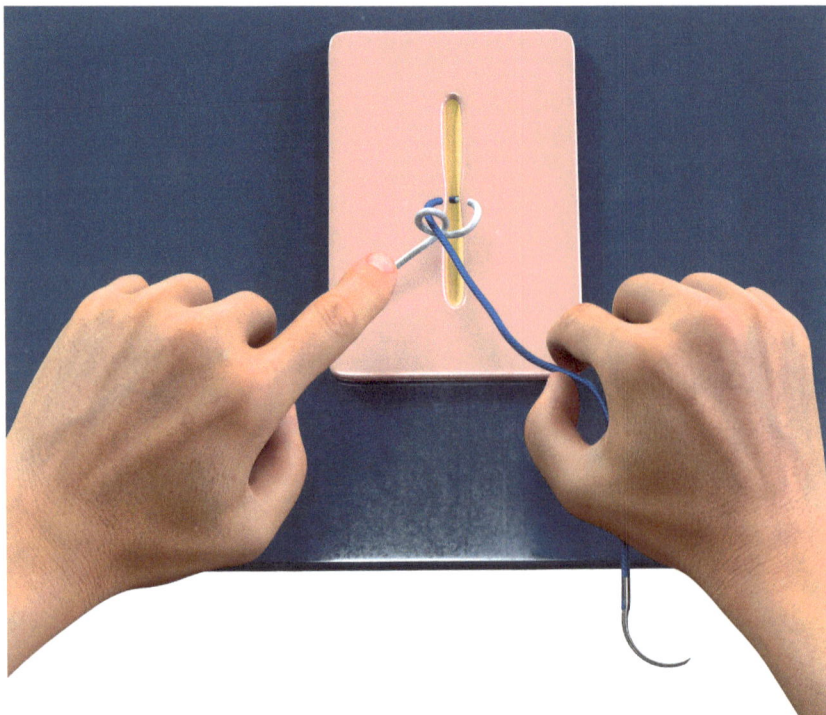

Step 6: Turn your left hand upwards, crossing the suture across your palm.

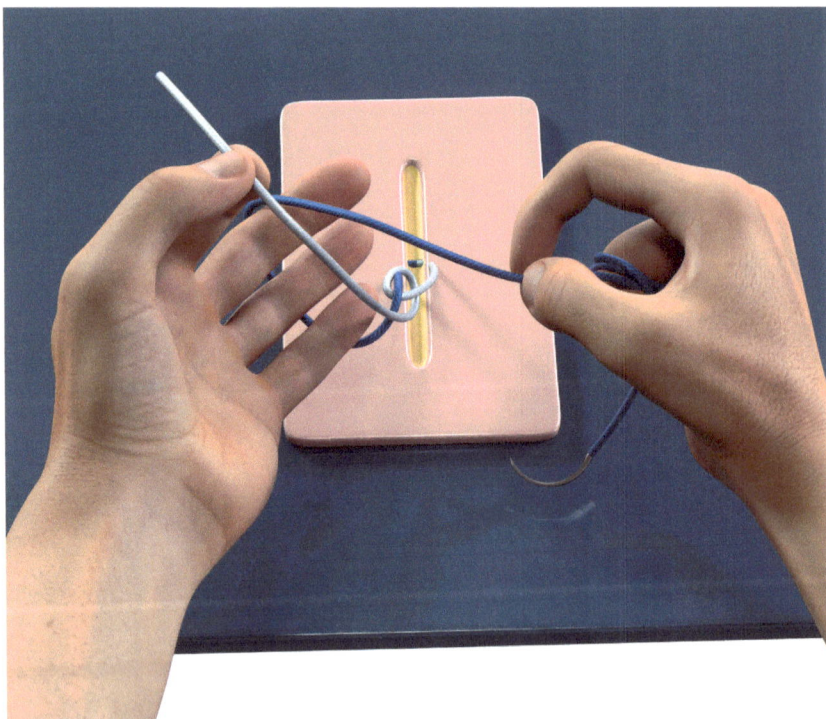

Step 7: Grasp the short end of the suture between your right middle and ring fingers and pull the end under the long end of the suture.

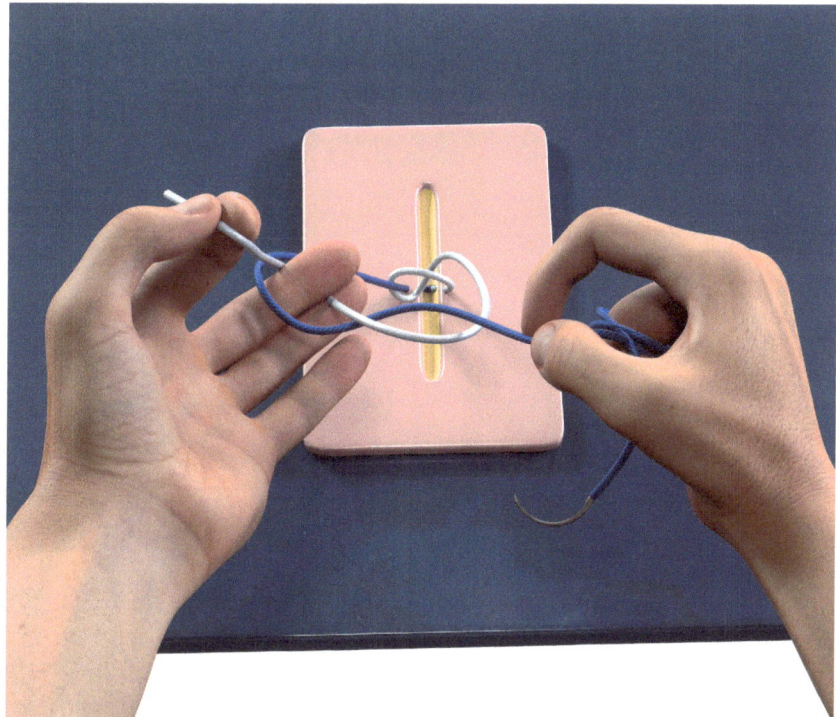

Step 8: Pull up on the long end of the suture again form a noose and slide this downwards.

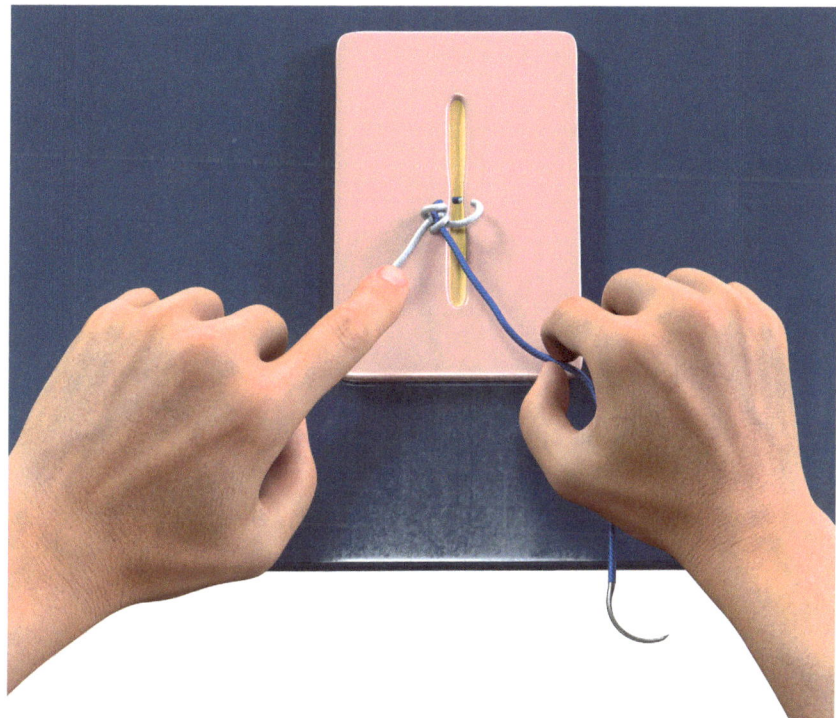

Step 9: Turn your left hand upwards and repeat the process of pulling the short end under the long end of the suture.

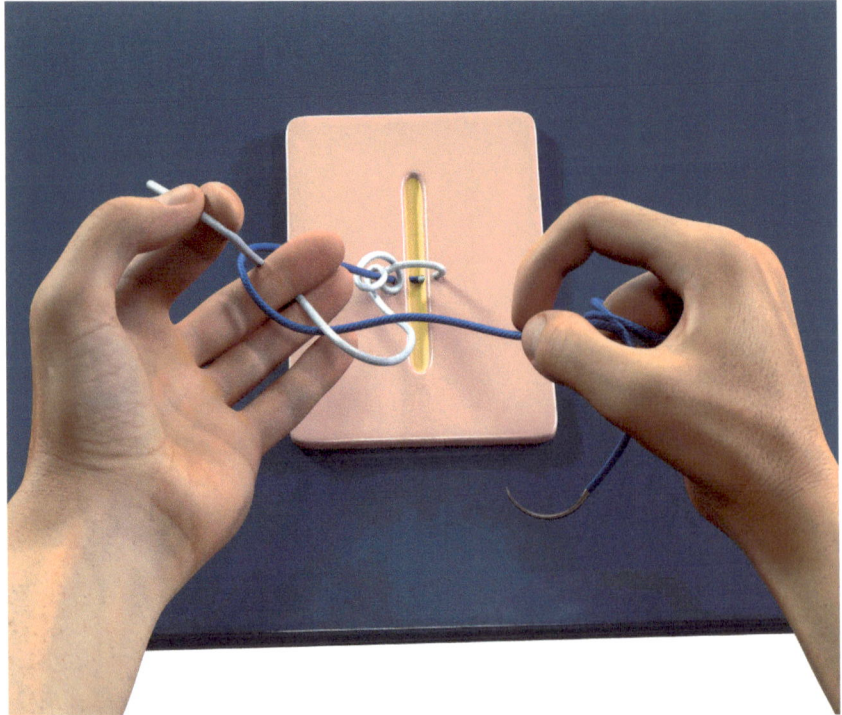

Step 10: Pull up on the long end of the suture and slide the noose downward to tighten the tissue.

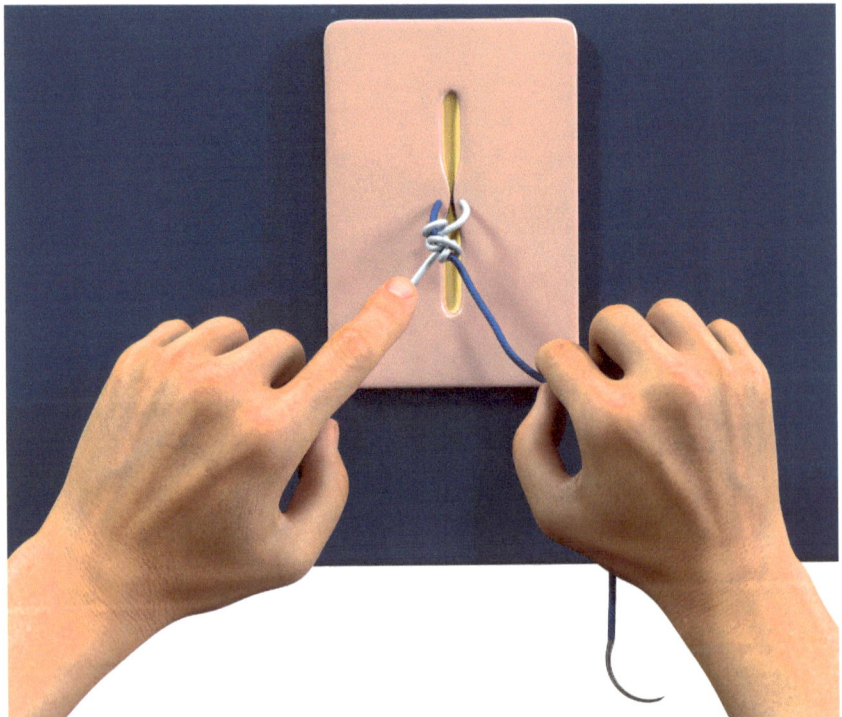

Step 11: Hook your left finger under the long end of the suture and use it to pull the short end under the long end of the suture.

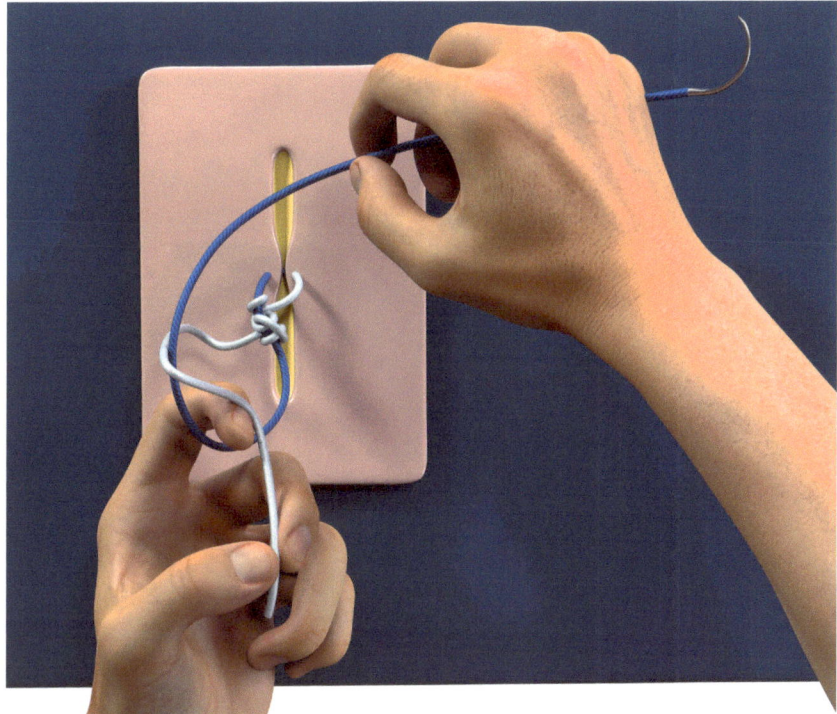

Step 12: Pull up on the short end of the suture and slide the long end down to tighten the tissue.

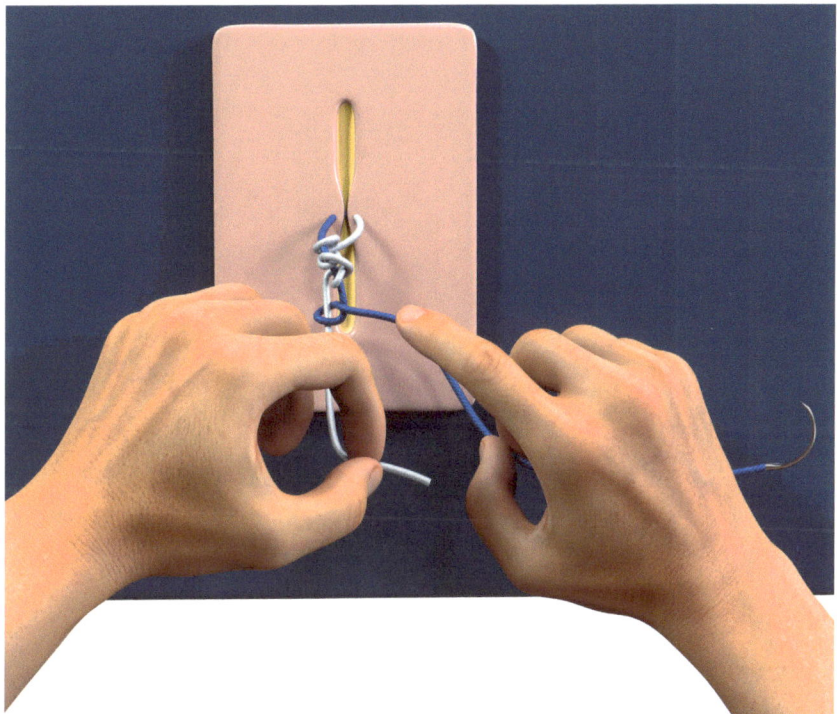

Step 13: Add an extra loop as in step one with your left hand and pull the suture down.

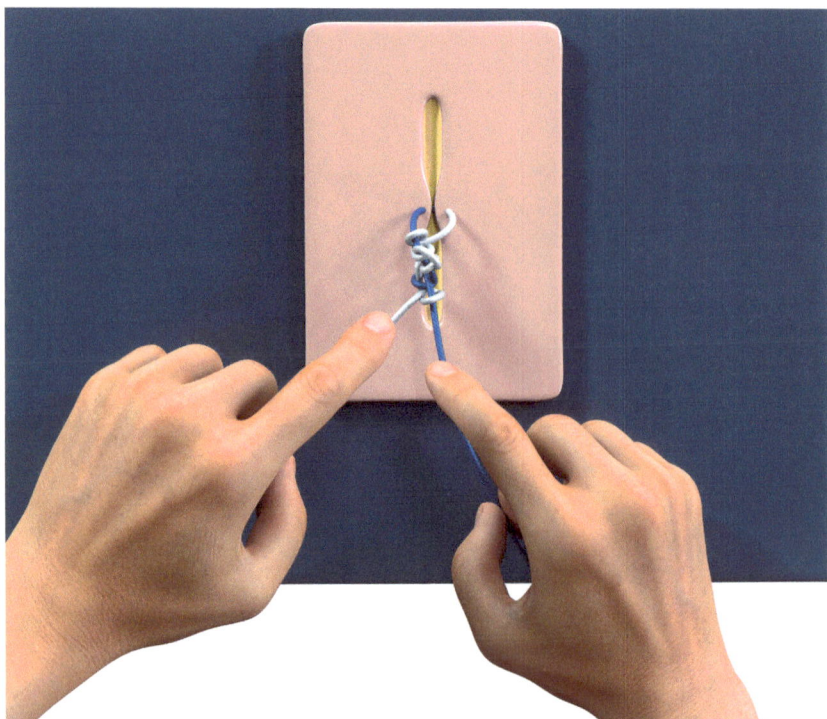

Critical aspects of knot tying

· After the first two knots are tied to appose the tissue, all subsequent throws should be done by pulling the short end of the suture parallel to the floor alternating away and towards you. Failure to do this will result in the knot failing to tie down flat, leading to slippage.

· Equally important is applying equal tension on both the short and long ends of the suture to prevent the formation of a noose. After the first two knots are tightened to secure the tissue, subsequent throws are done only to prevent slippage or unraveling. Avoid any tension on either end of the suture by lowering your hands until the throw hits the underlying knot. Never pull up hard with both ends of the suture. This leads to the locking of the knots, formation of air knots, or can pull the suture off or tear the tissue. A correctly tied knot should have tension in a straight line between the two ends of the suture, with the object to be ligated along that line.

· Start with the ends of the suture crossed, with the needle away from you and the short end towards you. Tie two-hand ties with the hand holding the needle end or one-hand knots with the hand holding the short end. Doing this prevents pulling the needle through the loop, causing potential injury, and assures that the initial knot ties down flat with your arms uncrossed.

· Developing kinesthetic memory is key to creating efficient and secure knots [51]. Practicing knot tying is the only way to learn.

Other important principles of knot tying

A study from the Mayo Clinic showed that poorly constructed knots were commonly tied even by experienced surgeons [1]. Recently, a group of surgeons from the University of Plymouth Hospitals looked at the result of failure to tie knots down flat, specifically by either tying knots down under tension or failure to cross the hands. They found that 20% of flat reef knots slipped, while 100% of knots tied under tension or with failure to cross hands slipped [52]. They concluded: "Meticulous technique of knot tying is essential for secure knots, appropriate tissue tension and the security of anastomosis and haemostasis affected."

· Fundamental principles of surgical technique include the use of sharp dissection and avoidance of burning and tearing of tissue. Always remember that the scalpel can be used as a dissecting tool to slice, press, punch, or shave - which is often gentler to tissue than other techniques. Knots tied in devitalized or ischemic tissue have a much lower chance of success.

· Choosing the best knot for a given surgical procedure depends on suture thickness, material, and coating and whether it will be subjected to high or cyclical loading. Other considerations are its local environment (in fat, moisture, etc.), the importance of knot profile or comfort of the suture, whether it needs to be placed through a trocar or in a small cavity, and whether some stretch of the loop is clinically important.

· Generally, since you will stitch forehand using your dominant hand, start the tie with sutures crossed and with the needle end in your dominant hand and the short end towards you, held by your non-dominant hand.

· The most common novice errors for two-handed tying are too much motion in the right hand, failure to maintain constant tension, hands too close to the knot, and failure to cross the hands.

· To ensure proper apposition of tissue, a noose is more reliable than a Surgeon's or Square knot for the first two throws when monofilament suture is used. A Granny noose resists back-slipping better than a Square noose. In a noose, unlike a knot pulled down flat, there should be very little tension on the short end of the suture. Tension on the short end tightens the knot and makes it more difficult to slip. Tension on the short end of the suture also results in no change in the length of the short end. The knot should be pushed down with the fingernail of the non-dominant index finger and only tightened when it is all the way down, to avoid upwards traction on tissue. Additional flat knots are required to ensure knot security and prevent loosening.

· Square and Granny knots can be converted to a noose, but a noose cannot reliably be converted back to a flat knot, so it is important that after the first two throws have been completed that subsequent throws are pulled down with equal tension and as flat knots .

· Knots deep down and in small spaces can be tied using alternating half hitches (Revo knot) or using ratcheting or self-locking knots.

Chapter 6: Instrument Ties and Microsurgical Knot Tying

Instrument tie: Surgeon's knot

Step 1: Instrument ties frequently use a Surgeon's knot for the first throw. Start with the needle holder in the "V" between the long end of the suture, the skin, and the short end of the suture.

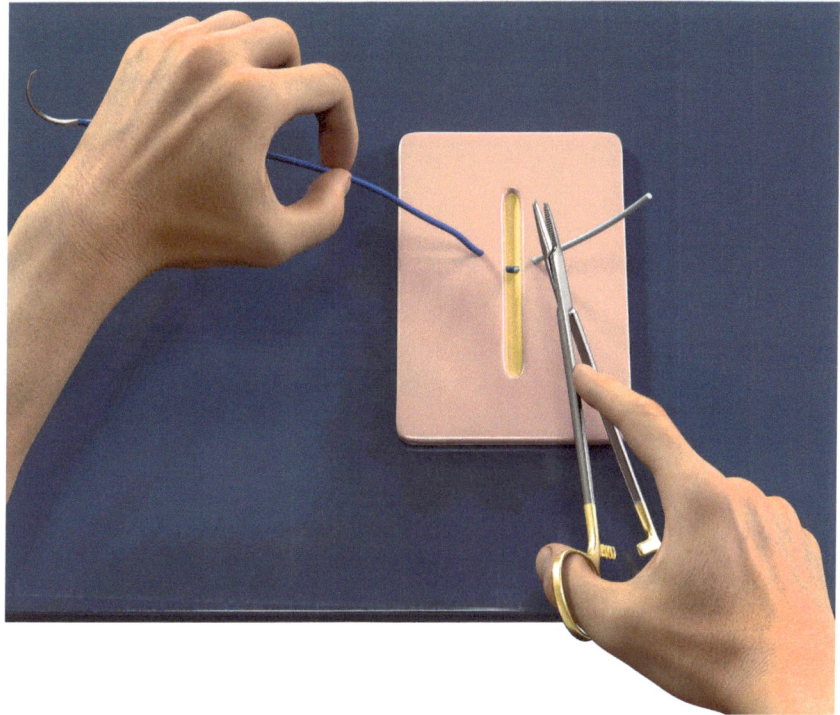

Step 2: Rather than twirling the needle holder around the suture, hold it still, and use your left hand to wrap the long end of the suture twice around the needle holder. Pull the long end of the suture slightly back towards you. Grasp the short end of the suture with the needle holder.

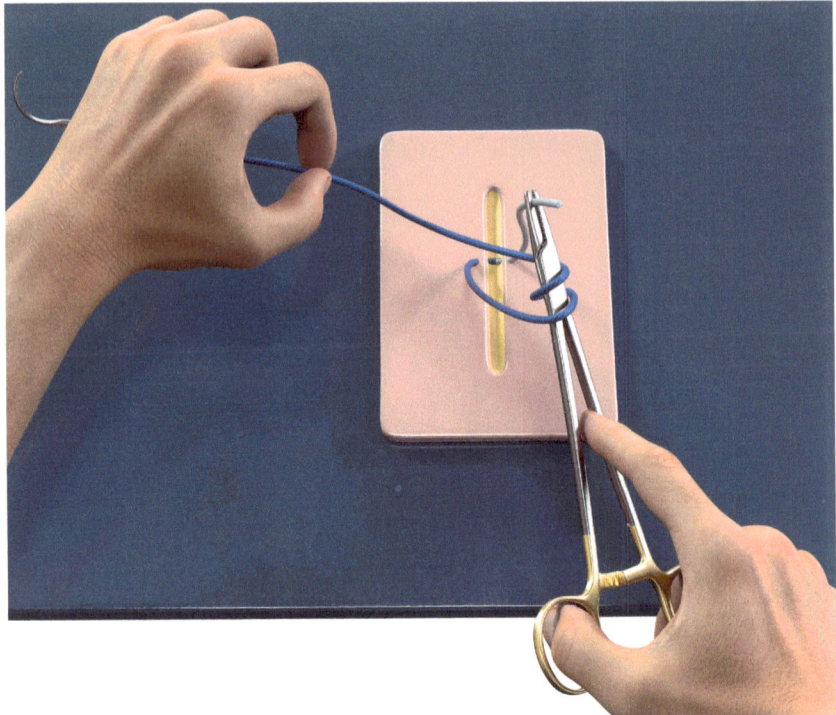

Step 3: Pull the needle holder slightly backward to allow the wrapped suture to fall off the tip. Pull the short end of the suture in the opposite direction from where it started (if it was to your right, pull it towards your left). If the tissue is under too much tension to hold, pull the short end back in the same direction as the long end (to lock it under the first throw).

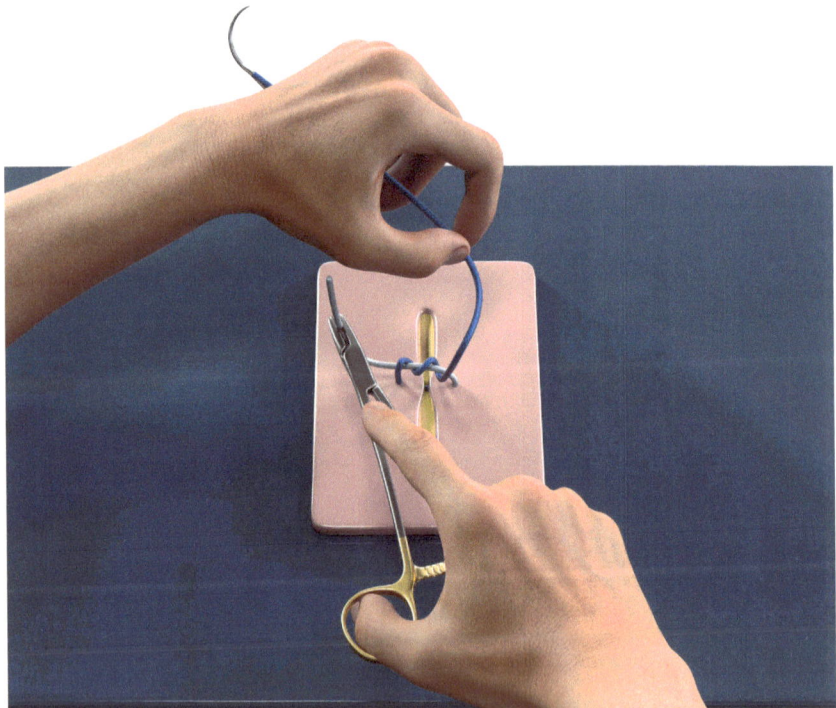

Step 4: Release the needle holder and hold its tip in the "V" between the short end, the knot, and the long end of the suture.

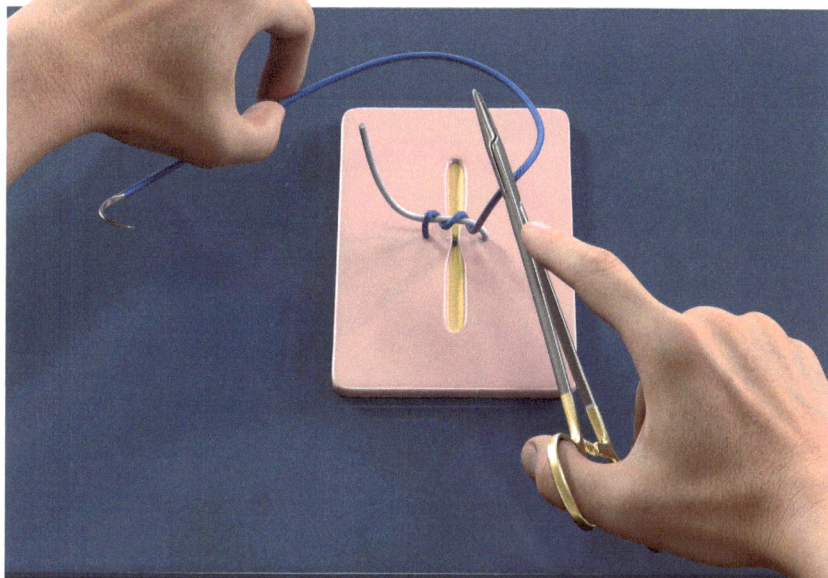

Step 5: Wrap the long end of the suture once around the needle holder and pull the long end slightly backward. Grasp the short end with the needle holder.

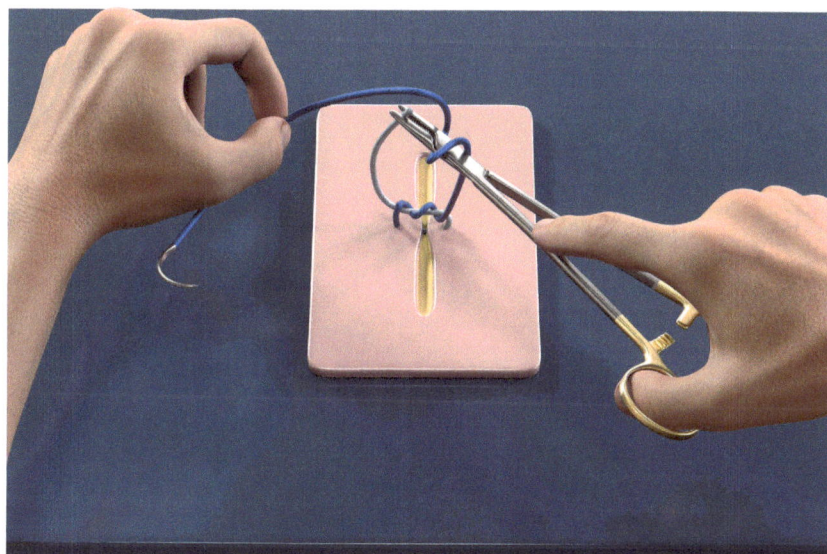

Step 6: Pull the long end of the suture to the left and the short end to the right to lay the knot down flat. Repeat steps 1-5, using single wraps around the needle holder, pulling the short end, and alternating to the left and right to ensure that the knot lies flat.

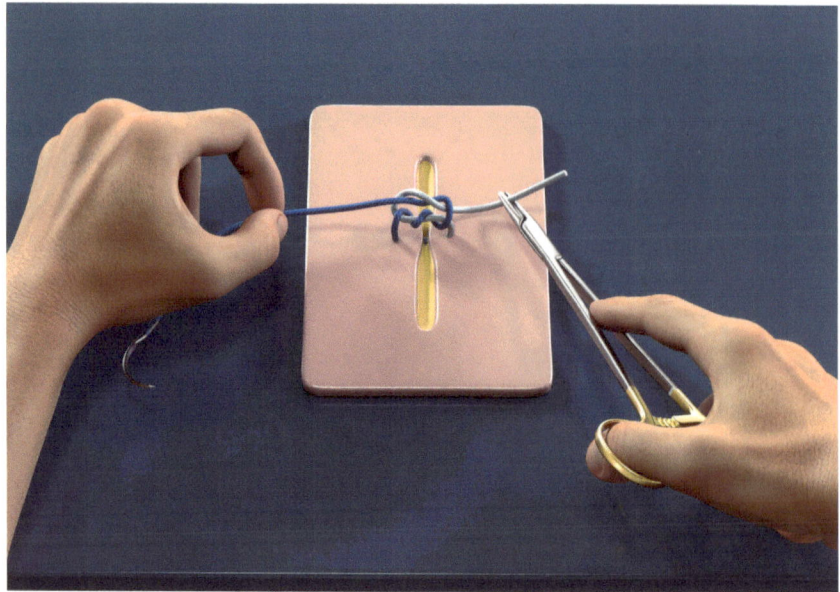

The Constrictor knot and its variants

A Constrictor knot is a reliable method for the ligation of vessels [25, 53]. The Constrictor knot is like a Clove Hitch except that an extra twist of the suture around itself is added at the end. In comparing the force required to slide a ligature along a rod, the Constrictor knot was shown to be superior to the Surgeon's knot and several other knots with Prolene, Vicryl, PDS, and Monocryl suture materials. It works best with monofilament suture.

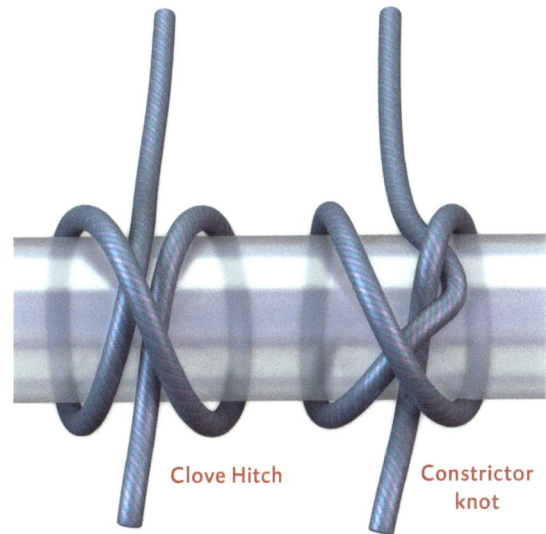

Clove Hitch   Constrictor knot

Instrument tying a Constrictor knot

The following method shows how an instrument can facilitate the ligation of a blood vessel using a Constrictor knot.

Step 1: Place the suture over the vessel and pull it back under and towards your right.

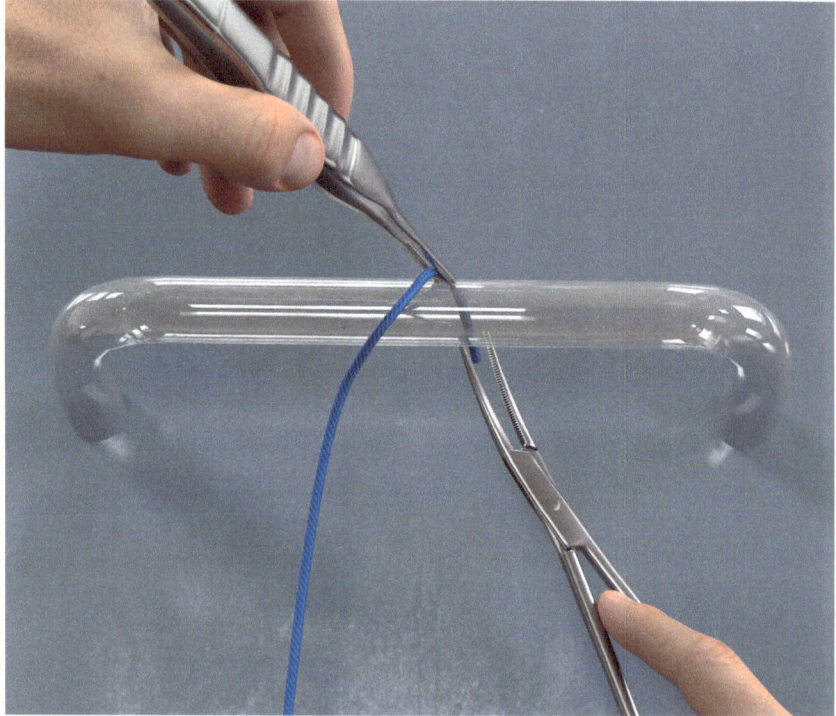

Step 2: Place the suture over the vessel, but this time pull it back under and towards your left.

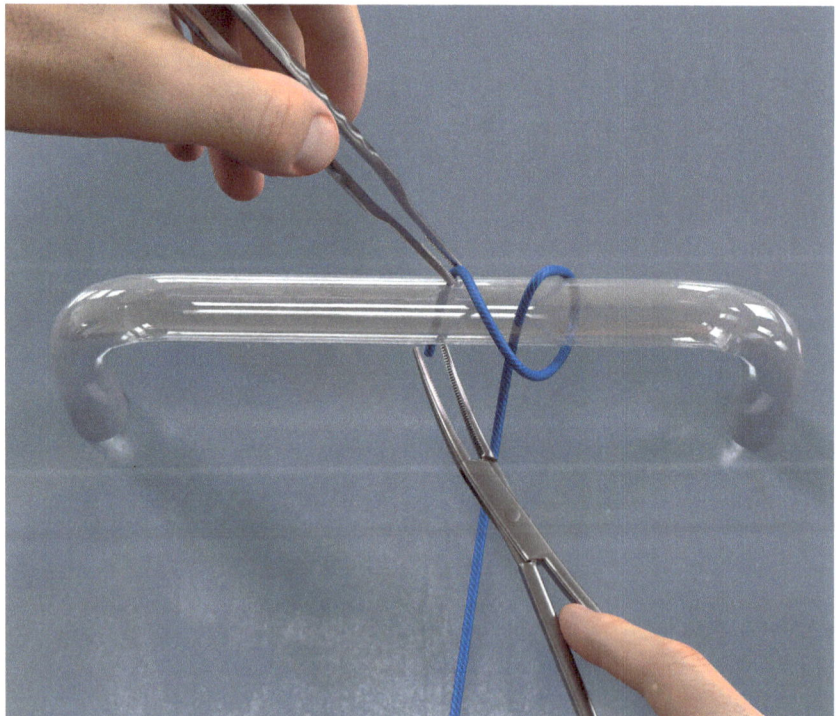

Step 3: Put the needle holder under the loop of the suture with tips pointing back towards your left.

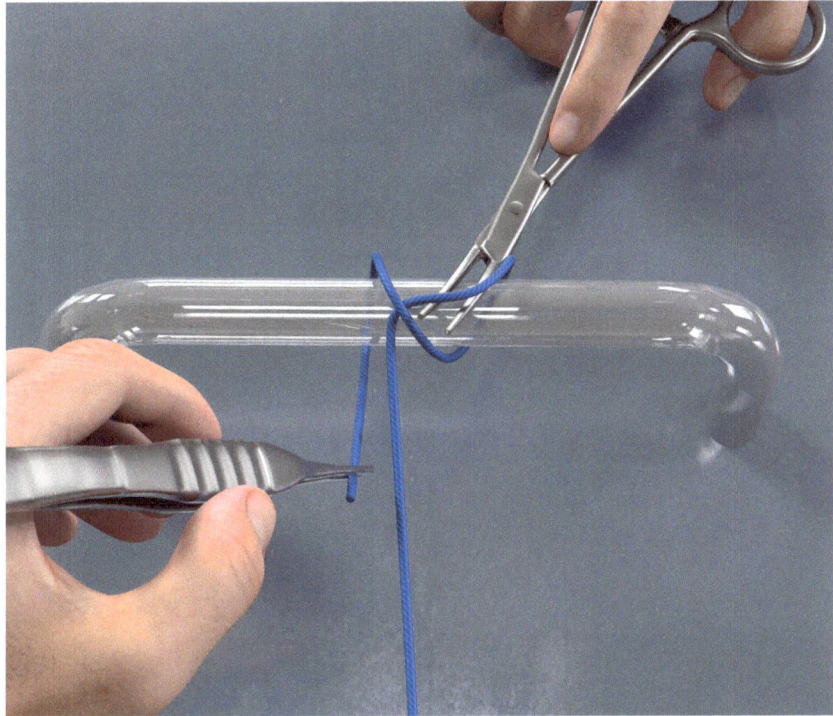

Step 4: Pass the tip of the needle holder over the suture's long end and grasp the suture's short end.

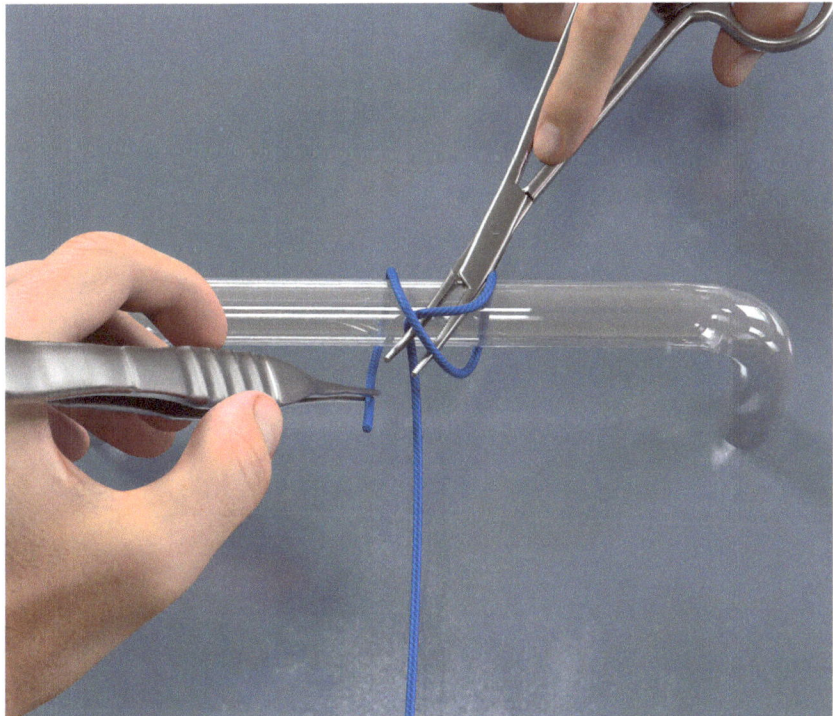

Step 5: Pull the short end of the suture away from you to tighten the Constrictor knot.

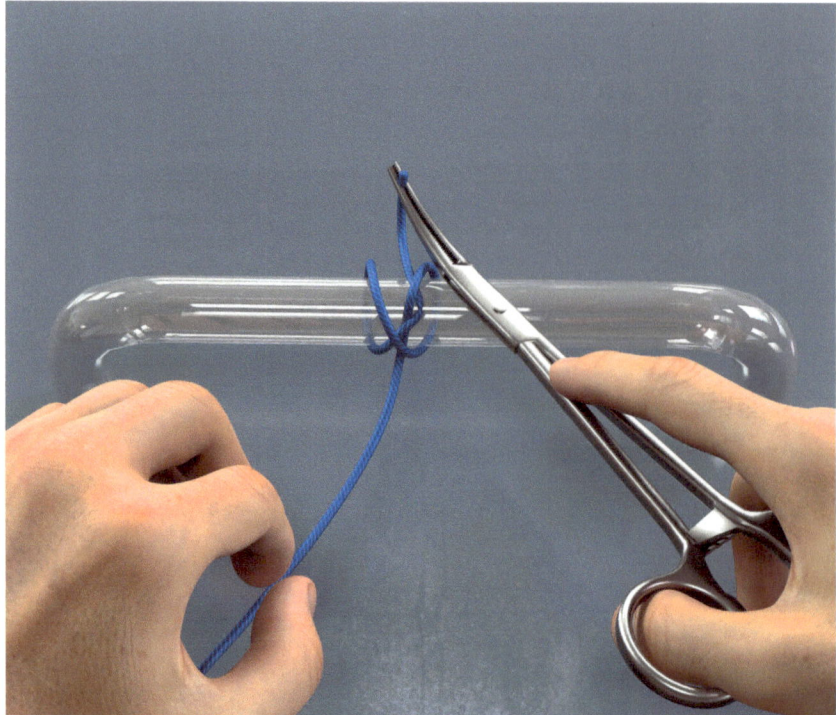

The Double Constrictor knot and Surgeon's variant

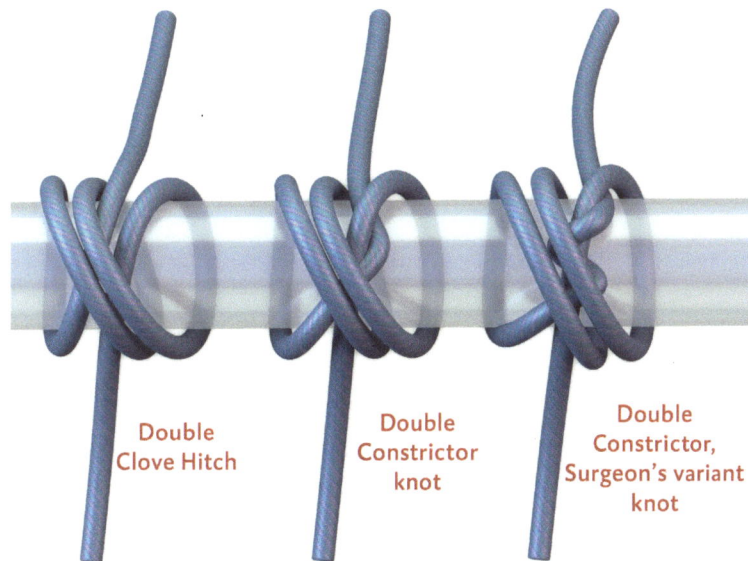

Double Clove Hitch

Double Constrictor knot

Double Constrictor, Surgeon's variant knot

The Double Constrictor knot and Surgeon's variant of the Double Constrictor are like a Double Clove hitch, except an extra twist or two is added at the end under the overriding sutures. These knots can secure a plastic tube in place, as they grip firmly and reduce the chance of the tube slipping through the suture. After hand tying the suture around the tube with a Double Constrictor or Surgeon's variant Double Constrictor, use the end with the needle to suture through the skin. Tie this to the other end of the suture with several Square knots to prevent loosening.

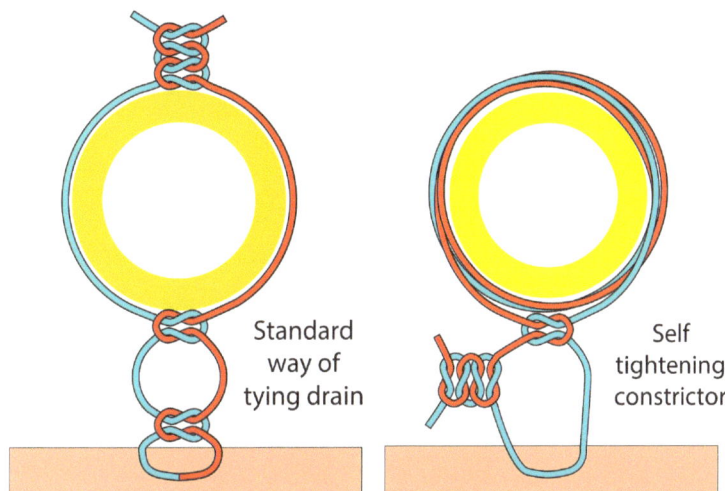

Standard way of tying drain

Self tightening constrictor

The standard way to tie in a drain with Square knots is not self-tightening and often loosens over time, leading to sliding of the drain.

Video of hand tying Constrictor knot:
https://www.youtube.com/watch?v=T8ixCl9dtC4

Video of hand tying Double Constrictor knot:
https://www.youtube.com/watch?v=CZzkMeAUiSc

Microsurgical Knot tying

Microsurgical knot tying is similar to the previously described instrument ties. However, since one is tying very small suture (often 10-0) with magnification ranging from 3X to 40X power, care must be done to avoid excessive movement of your hands, and tying is almost completely done by sight rather than by feel. It helps to rest your arms on a soft surface to minimize motion.

Tying with two jeweler's forceps

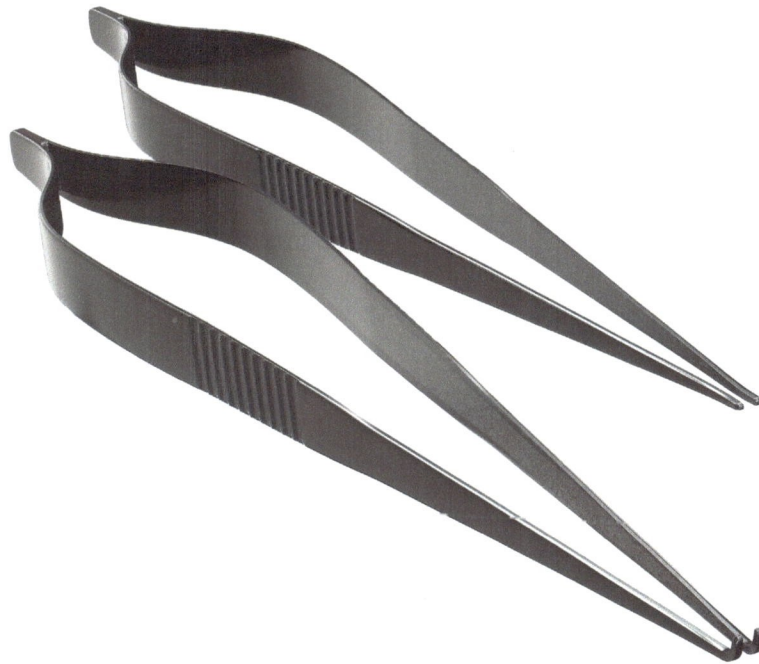

Figure 6.1: Two Jeweler's Forceps

The following illustrations show suture that is larger than would appear under the microscope, but are used to show the conformation of the knot.

Step 1: With curved jeweler's forceps in your left hand and straight jeweler's forceps in your right hand, pull the suture enough to leave about a 3 mm tail. The long end of the suture should be held about three times further from the tissue than the short end, with the long end directed away from the short end. During the entire knot tying process, do not release the forceps holding the long end.

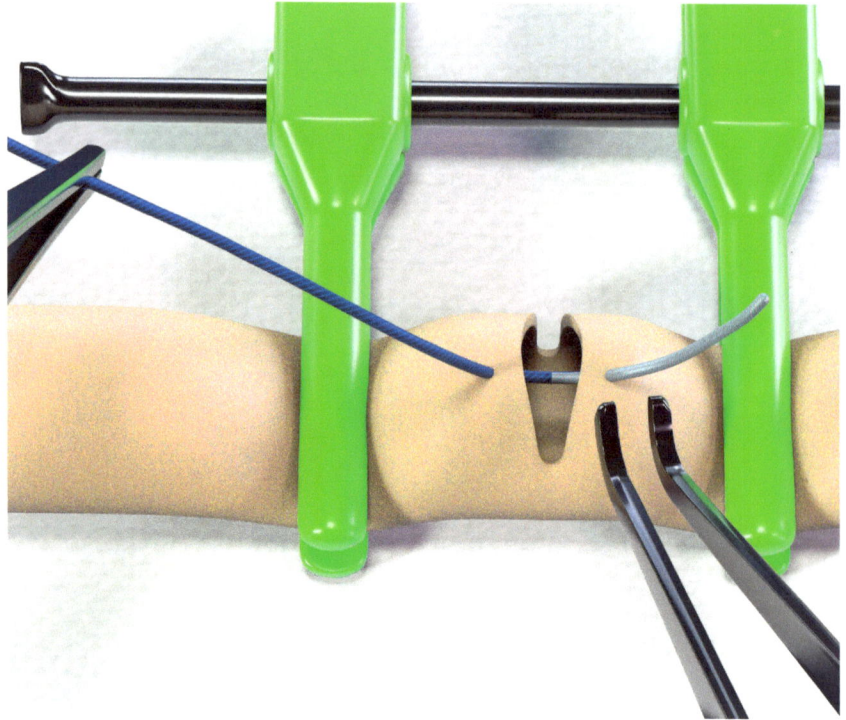

Note: It is important not to pick up the long end in such a way that the long end points towards the short end. That will make it almost impossible to form the loop necessary to tie a knot.

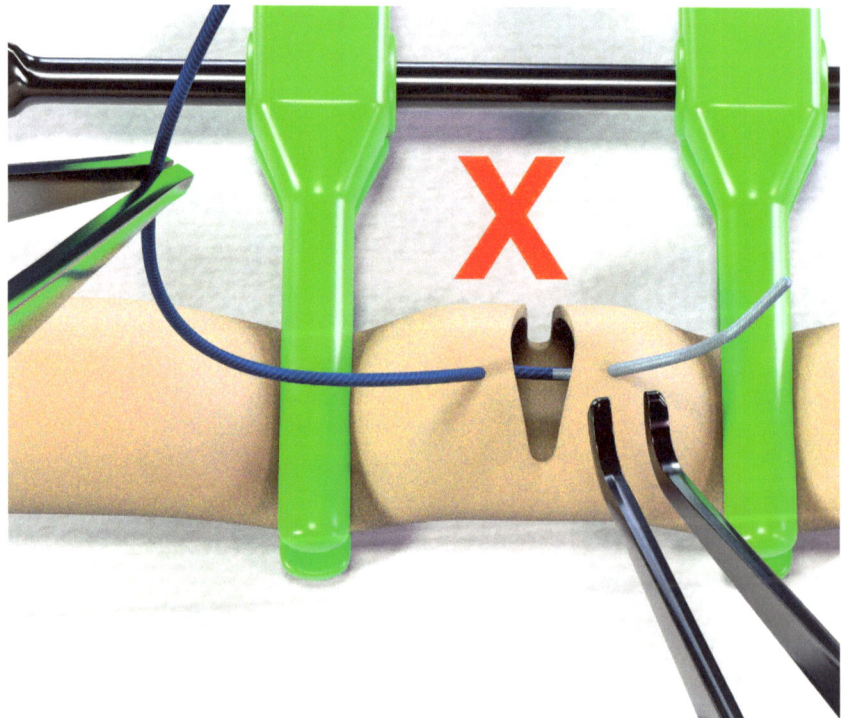

Unless one intention-
ally wishes to tie a
Granny Knot, do not
place the forceps in
your right hand outside
the "V" between the
long and short ends of
the suture. Wrapping
the long end around
the suture placed
outside the "V" will
be more difficult and
results in a non-Square
knot.

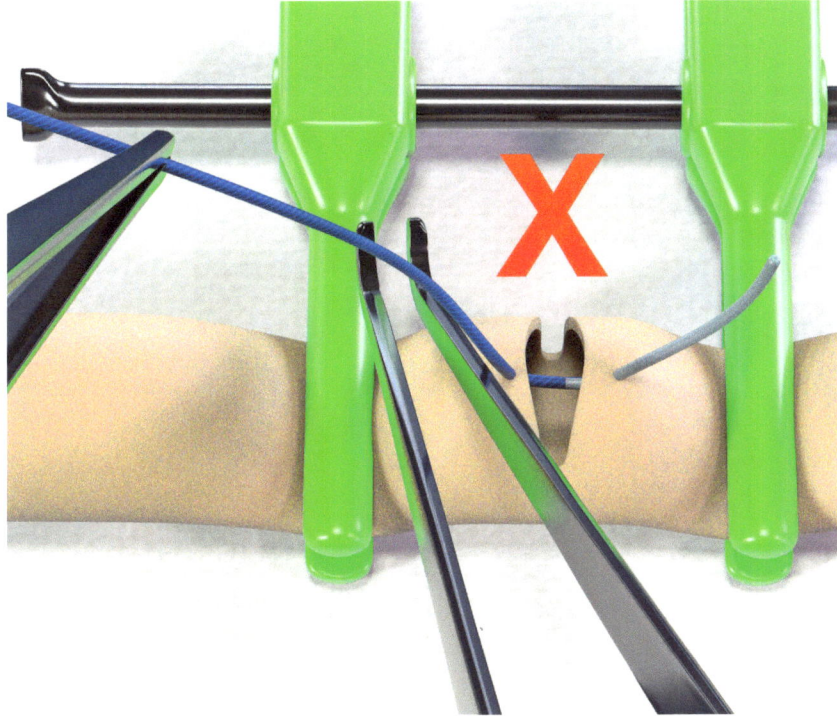

Step 2: Pull the long
end of the suture to-
wards the short end
with the forceps in
your left hand, and
move the jeweler's
forceps in your right
hand towards the left
to begin to form a loop.

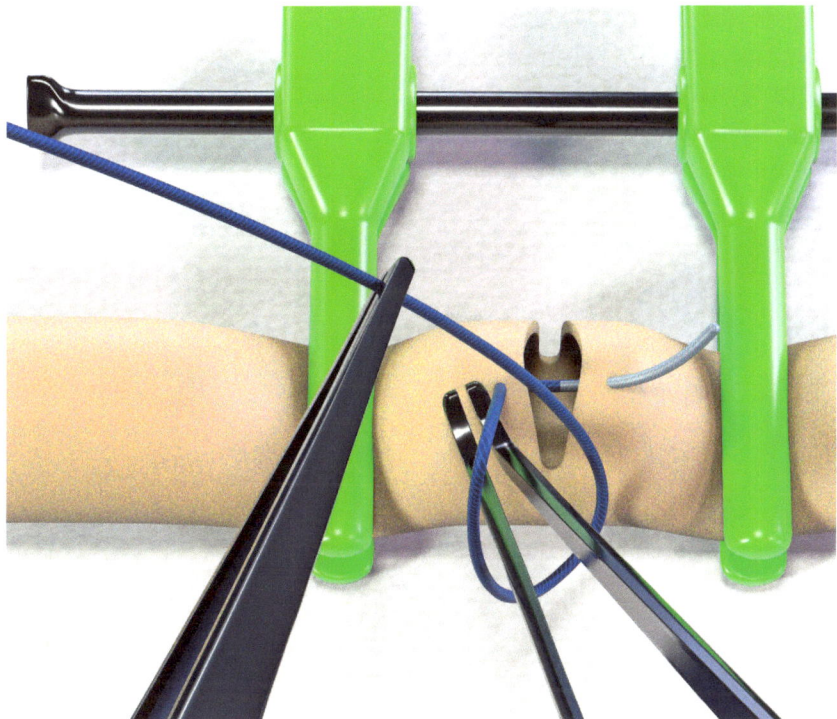

Step 3: Pull the suture in your left forceps towards you and downwards to complete the loop around the right forceps, turning the forceps in your right hand to point towards the short end of the suture.

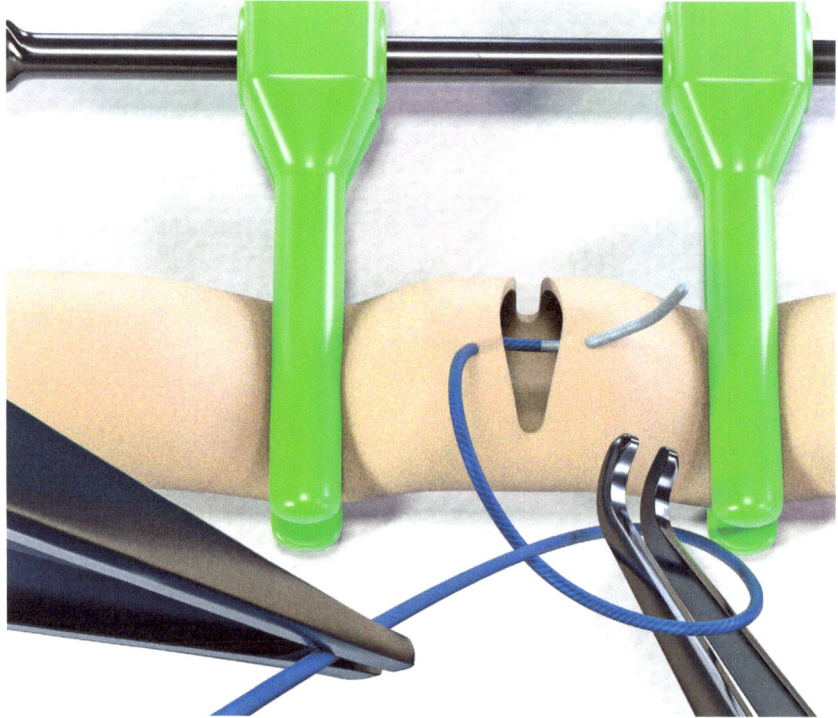

Step 4: Grasp the short end of the suture with the forceps in your right hand, ensuring the tips are directed parallel to the short end.

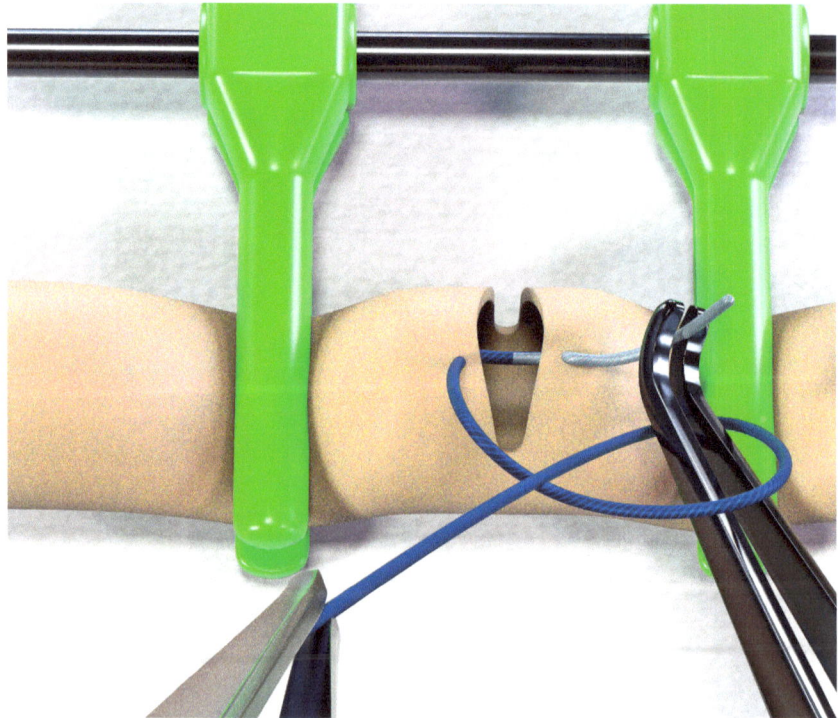

Note: If the tips of the forceps in your right hand are not directed parallel to the short end, it will be difficult to grasp the short end correctly.

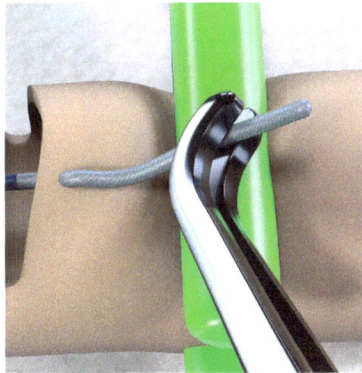

Parallel

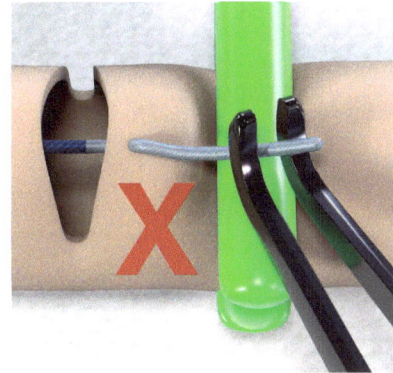

Not Parallel

Step 5: Pull the short end to your left and the long end to your right, forming an overhand knot.

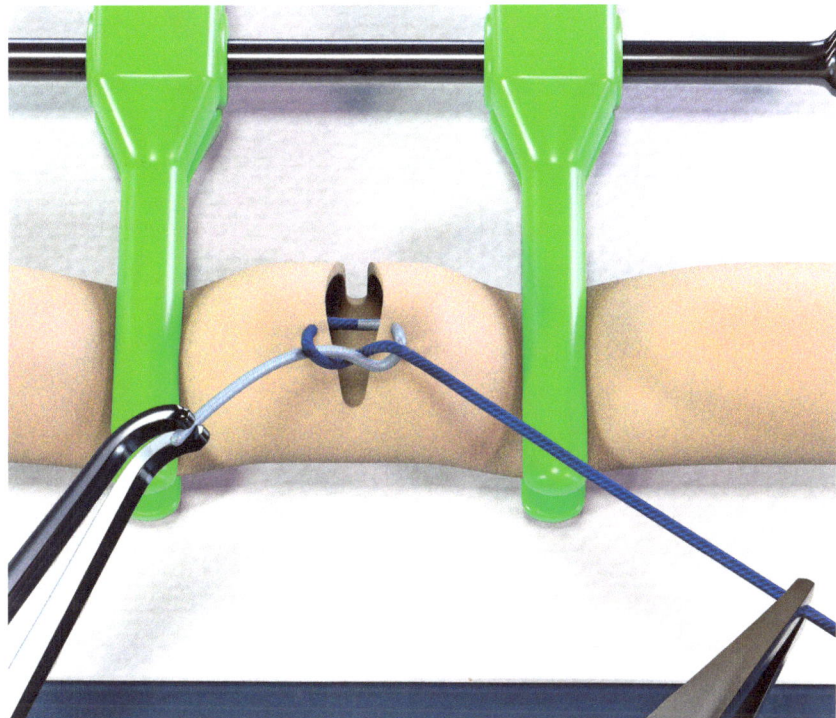

Step 6: Without letting go of the long end of the suture, wrap it around the jeweler's forceps in your right hand.

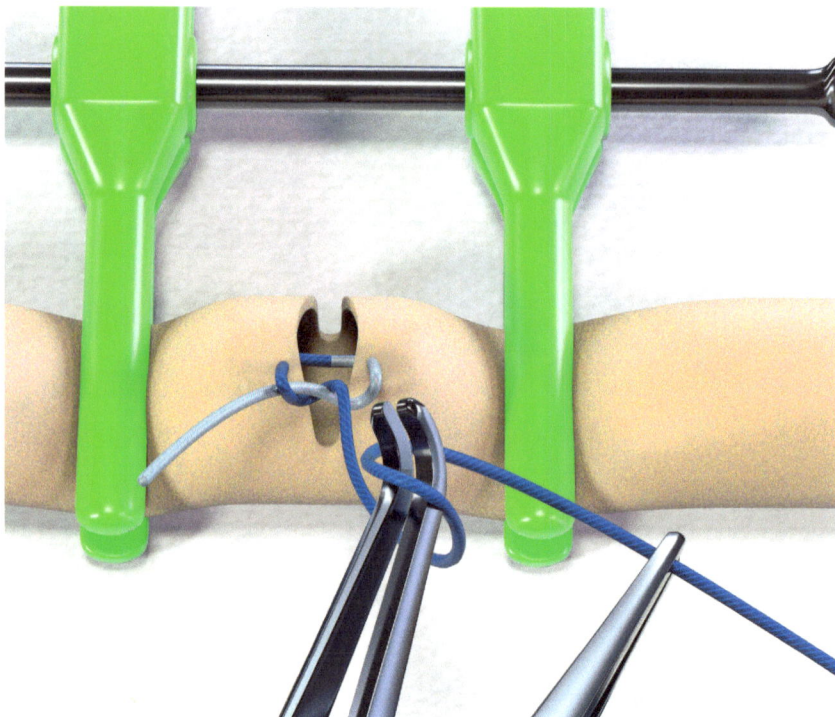

Step 7: Grasp the short end of the suture with the jeweler's forceps in your right hand.

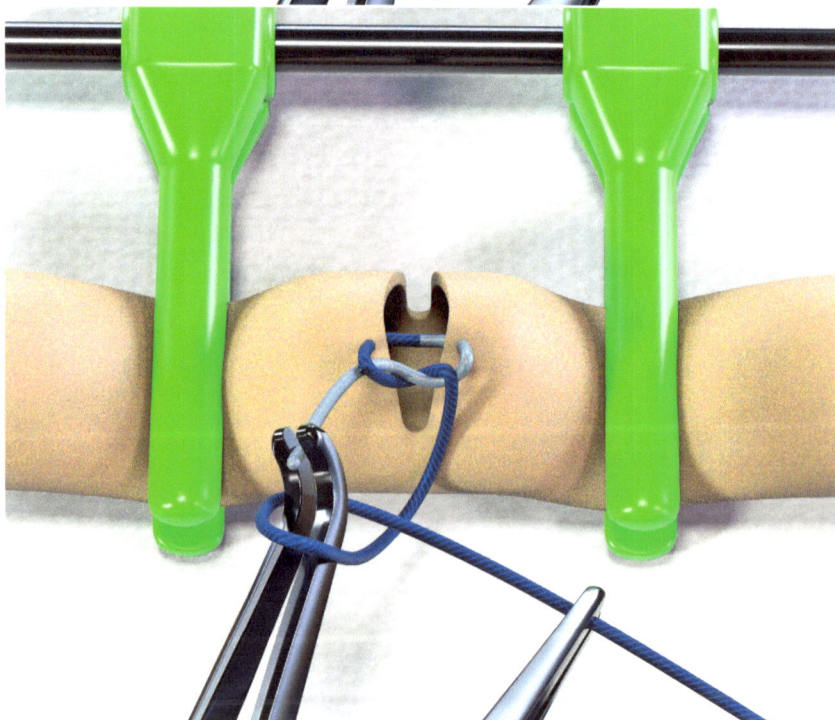

Step 8: Holding the short end in place, pull the long end to your right, converting the knot to a noose to approximate the tissue.

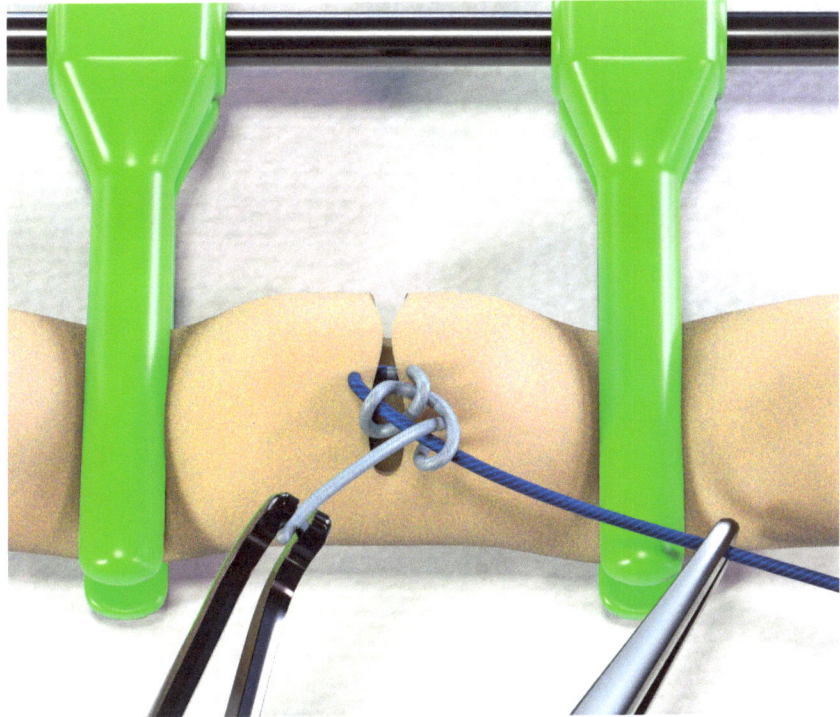

Add additional overhand knots, repeating the same steps as before, but pulling the short end alternating to the right and left, so that the knots lie flat.

Tying with jeweler's forceps and a Castroviejo needle driver

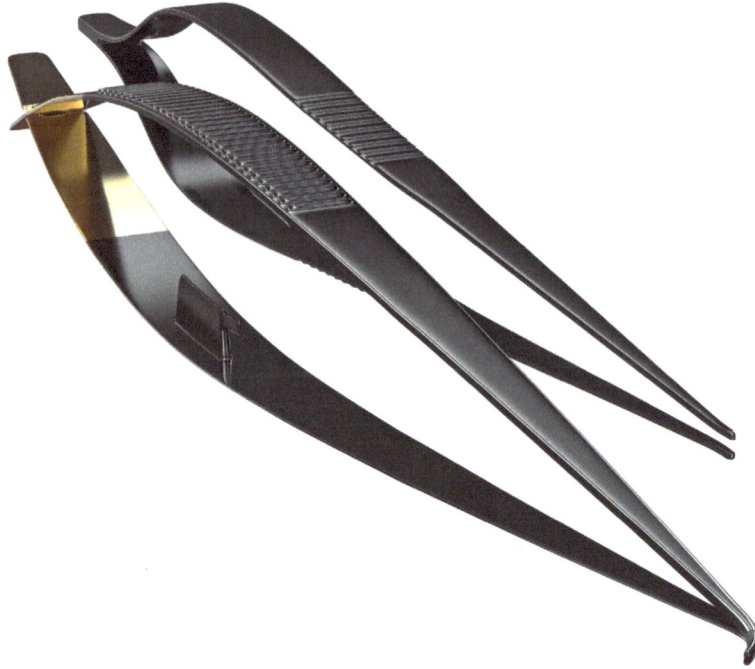

Figure 6.2: Microsurgical Instruments

The following method shows how to tie a knot if one is using a Castroviejo needle driver and you wish to hold the needle driver so the tip is pointed in the opposite direction from the jeweler's forceps. This may be advantageous if the sutured area faces towards and away from you, rather than right to left. If the tip of needle holder is pointed in the same direction as the tip of the jeweler's forceps, the method for tying a knot would be the same as that used with two jeweler's forceps.

Step 1: With jeweler's forceps in your left hand and a microsurgical suture holder in your right hand, pull the suture enough to leave about a 3 mm tail. The long end of the suture should be held about three times further away from the tissue than the short end.

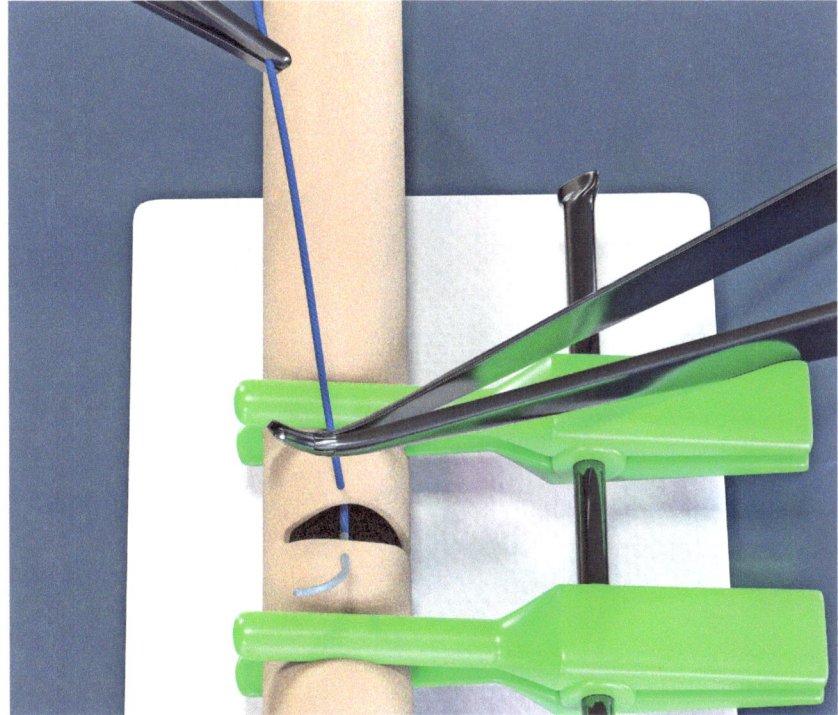

Step 2: Pass the long end of the suture around the tip of the needle holder so as to form a loop and push the long end of the suture slightly away from you to prevent it from coming off the needle holder.

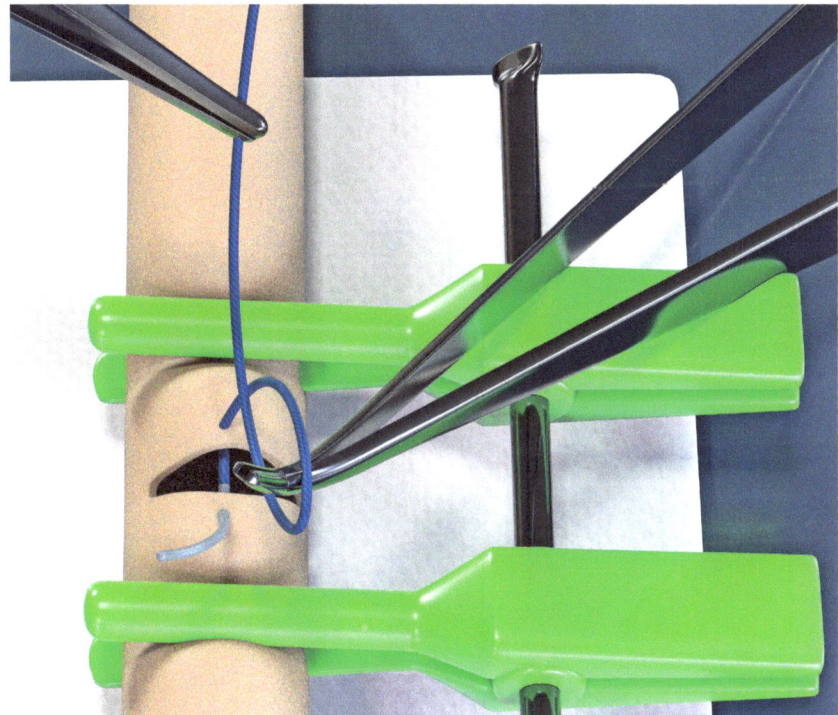

Step 3: Grasp the short end of the suture with the needle holder.

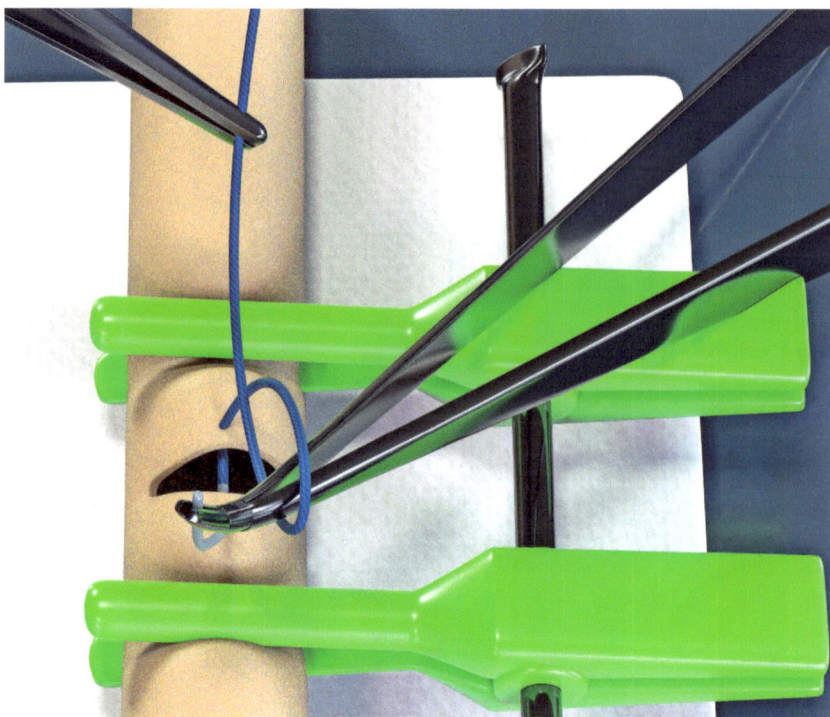

Step 4: Tie the first throw down flat by pulling the short end away from you and the long end towards you.

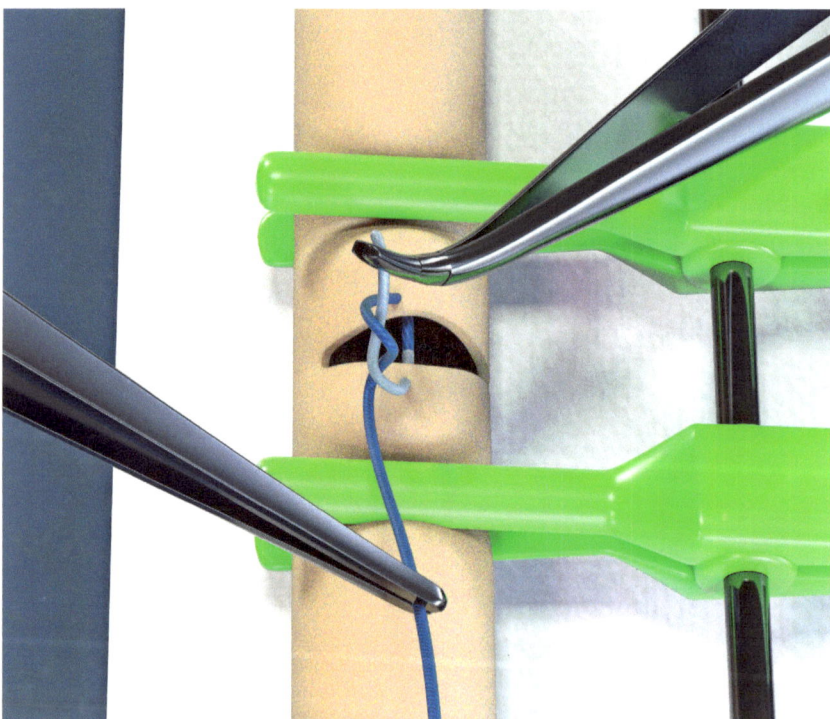

Step 5: Using the jeweler's forceps in your left hand, make a second loop of suture around the tip of the needle holder.

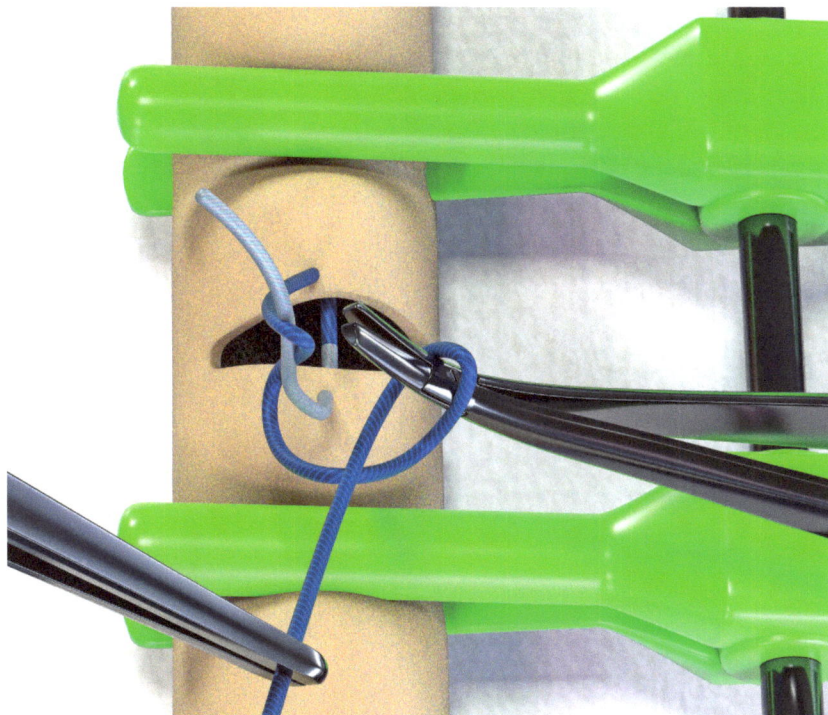

Step 6: Holding the short end in place, pull on the long end to convert the knot to a noose and pull it down tightly to oppose the sutured tissue.

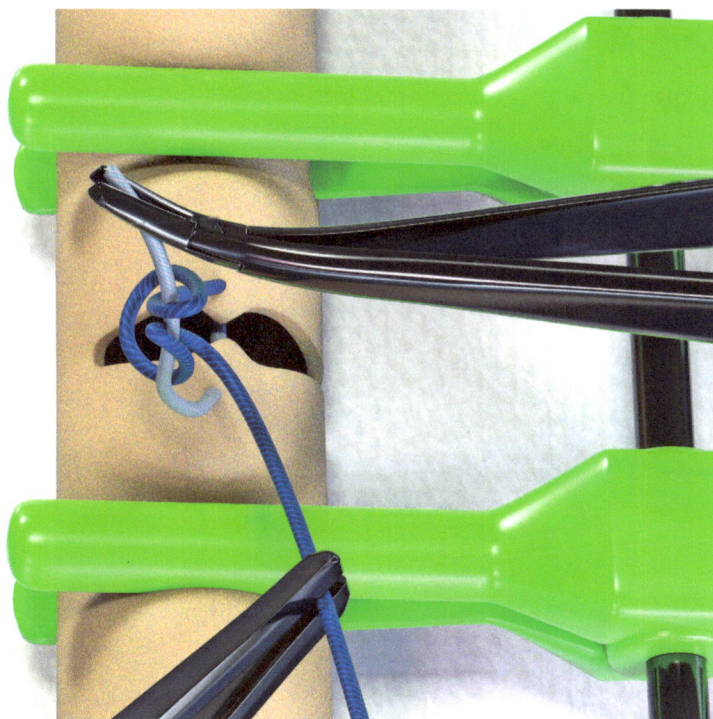

Step 7: Tie subsequent throws down flat by alternating pulling the short end of the suture towards and away from you.

After completing the knot, trim the short end and then cut the long end.

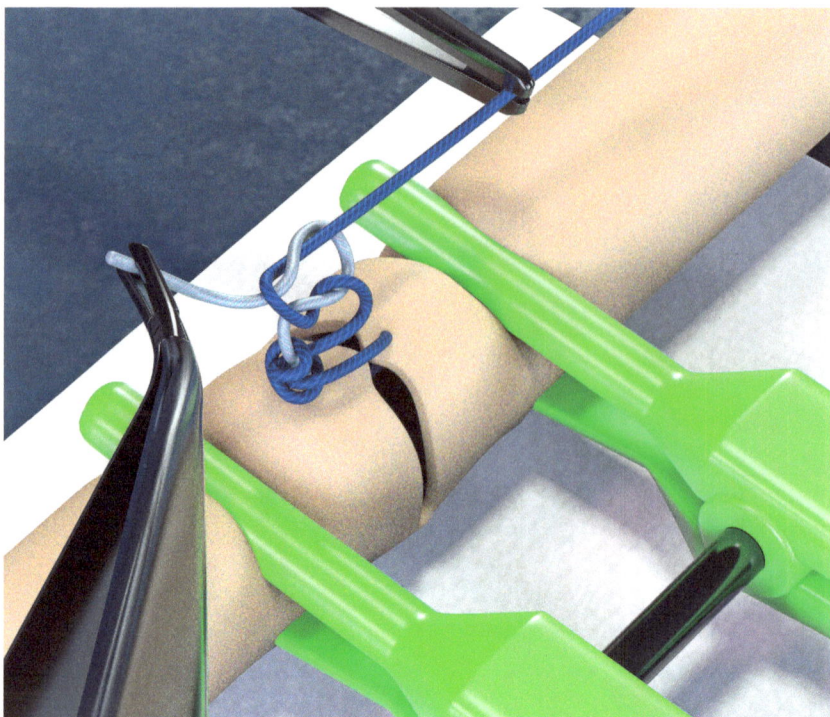

Videos of technique:

https://www.youtube.com/watch?v=FzQ3RNjreg4

https://www.youtube.com/watch?v=3tDYU3f1XfY

Chapter 7: Knots with Asymmetric Tension

The knots at the beginning or end of running suture have asymmetric tension. The security of these knots differs from knots with symmetric forces acting on them.

Aberdeen knot

The Aberdeen knot is similar to crocheting and was developed from the Highwayman's Hitch. It is used to end a continuous suture, such as a running subcuticular or fascial suture. Compared to Square knots, it is less likely to break [23, 54]. The most secure version of the Aberdeen knot consists of creating three loops and then pulling the suture twice through the end loop [55]. In their 2002 Basic Surgical Skills Course, the Royal College of Surgeons recommended using six loops and one turn, but tests show no benefit from more than three loops. Breaking strength may be improved by pulling the suture twice rather than once through the terminal loop.

   The Aberdeen knot has high security as long as the last strand is pulled through the loop and is long. All the loops underneath can unravel if it is short and pulls back through the final loop. The method of tying the Aberdeen knot for subcuticular closures can also be used for fascial closure. A recent paper proposed ending a continuous suture placed laparoscopically using the Aberdeen knot [56].

Step 1: Start by lifting the loop just before the end of the suture with your left hand, holding the needle end of the suture with your right hand.

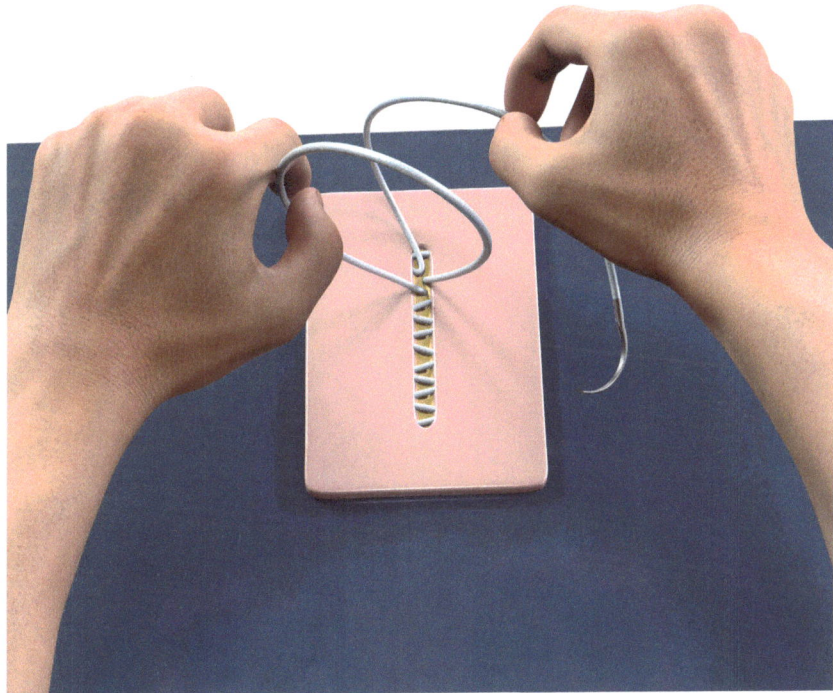

Step 2: With your left hand, grab the distal suture through the first loop and pull it through to form a second loop.

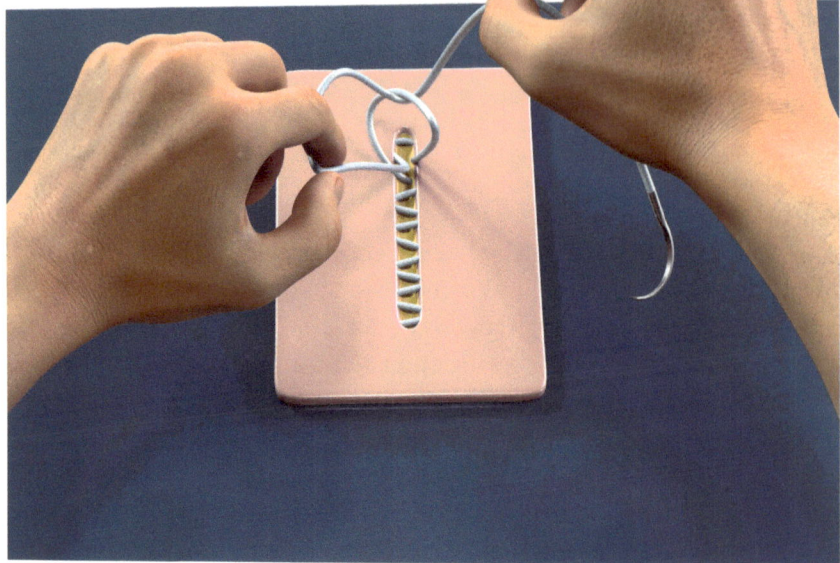

Step 3: Pull on the second loop to snug down the first loop.

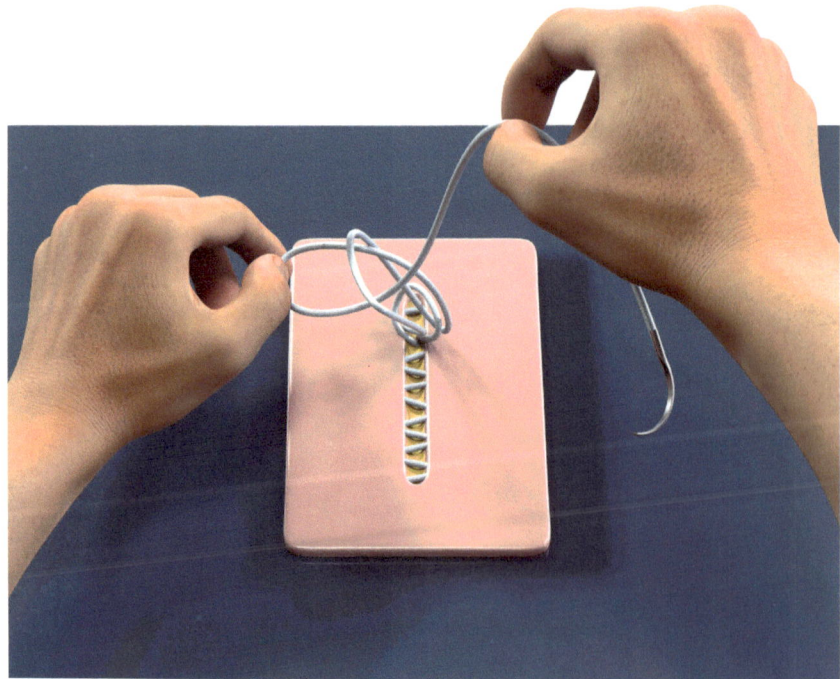

Step 4: Repeat steps 2 and 3 two more times. Pull the needle end of the suture through the loop once or twice and pull up on the needle end to pull down the last loop. Using the needle holder, pass the needle from deep in the tissue to exit through the skin away from the incision. Cut off the suture at the skin exit site.

Using two sutures

The best way to end a running suture is to tie a standard flat knot somewhere in the middle after running a second suture in the opposite direction. This avoids the problem of knot security when a loop is tied to a single strand of the suture. Of course, this requires three knots: one at each end of the sutures and a third in the middle. This is the recommended way of closing fascia after a laparotomy and generally the preferred method for laparoscopy.

Loop to single end tie over the top of suture

A standard method of ending a continuous suture is to tie the terminal loop, as if it were a single strand, to the end of the suture using traditional one-handed or two-handed tying techniques. However, this technique requires lots of throws for security, and the resulting knot can stick upwards towards the skin and eventually result in extrusion or suture abscess. Tying a loop to a single suture as a Square knot is common but is less secure than using an Aberdeen knot [54].

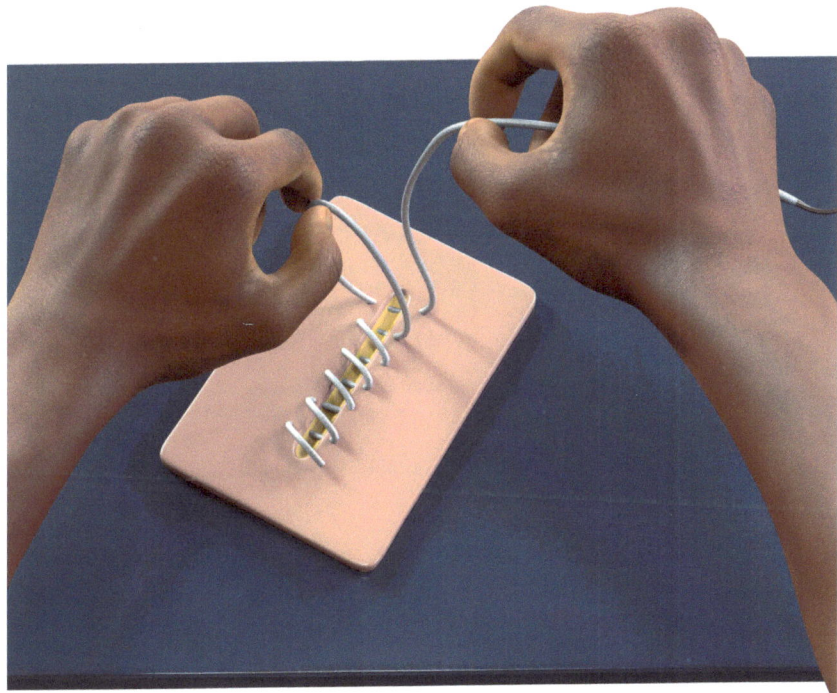

Some surgeons reverse the direction of the last loop (forehand to backhand), which results in a neater knot, where the loop and end of the suture are at opposite sides of the tissue being approximated.

Loop to single end tie under suture

A better way to tie a loop to a single strand is to choose a loop on the underside of the suture and run the needle down on the final pass so that the tied knot sticks downward rather than upwards. If the loop is too short, an accessory suture can be placed through the terminal loop to make it easier to tie down.

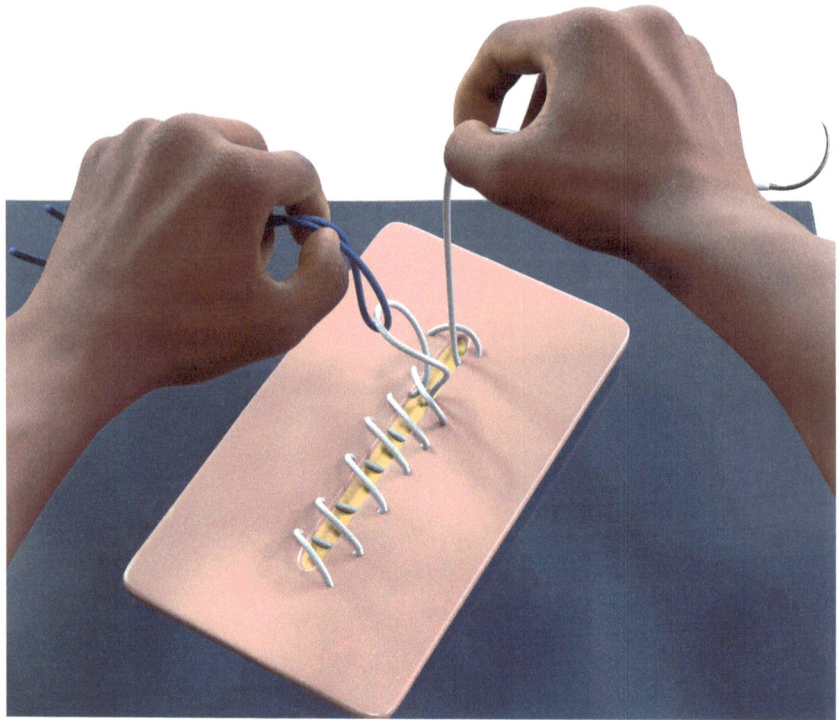

Using interrupted in place of continuous suture

Continuous sutures distribute tension better than interrupted sutures and are preferred for fascial closure. However, continuous sutures can bunch tissue and are usually avoided for small vascular or biliary anastomoses. For skin closures, using interrupted absorbable sutures has several advantages over a continuous subcuticular closure. It results in better apposition and more precise alignment of skin edges and creates less ischemia. You can remove single sutures postoperatively without disrupting the entire closure if a hematoma or subcutaneous abscess needs to be drained.

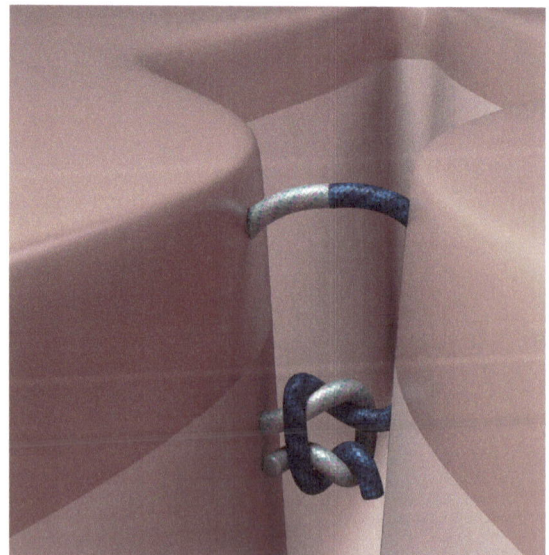

The downside to the placement of interrupted subcutaneous sutures is that the knots can extrude through the skin, resulting in scarring and suture abscesses. This risk can be minimized by suturing upside down so that the knot lies deep in the subcutaneous tissue. Monofilament sutures have less reactivity and a lower chance of harboring bacteria than braided sutures, but the knots needed for security are bulkier. It is important to tie the least bulky knot that ensures knot security to minimize the risk of suture extrusion through the skin. The cut ends should be kept short.

Chapter 8: Extracorporeal and Arthroscopic Knots

Extracorporeal knots are knots tied outside the body and slid into place through trocars using an open or closed knot pusher. Closed knot pushers can push and pull the knot without the suture slipping off the instrument but cannot be placed on the suture after it is inside the body. Unlike intracorporeal techniques, extracorporeal knots can be placed through a single access port.

Using a knot pusher for counter-traction

The method taught to general surgical residents in the Fundamentals of Laparoscopic Surgery curriculum uses a knot pusher to push down the suture after performing a one-handed or two-handed knot outside the body [57, 58]. If an open knot pusher is used, the knots can be pulled down flat by pulling away alternating sides of the suture with each throw.

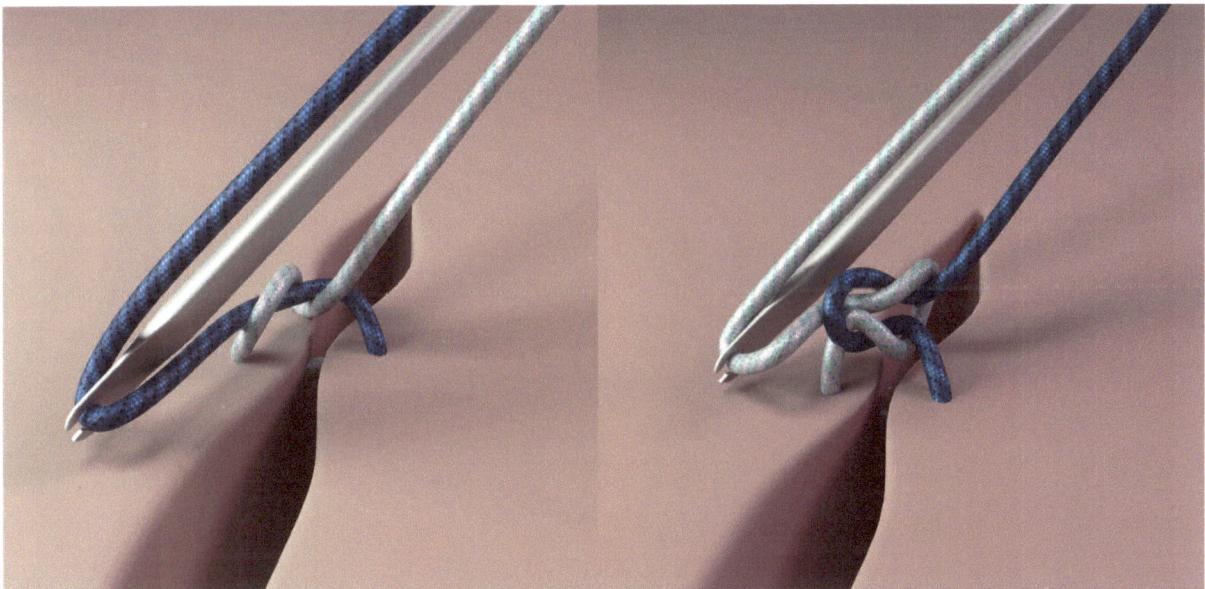

If a closed knot pusher is used, it can be left on the non-suture end, and successive knots can be placed using a one-hand technique. However, doing so may lead to a noose rather than flat knots.

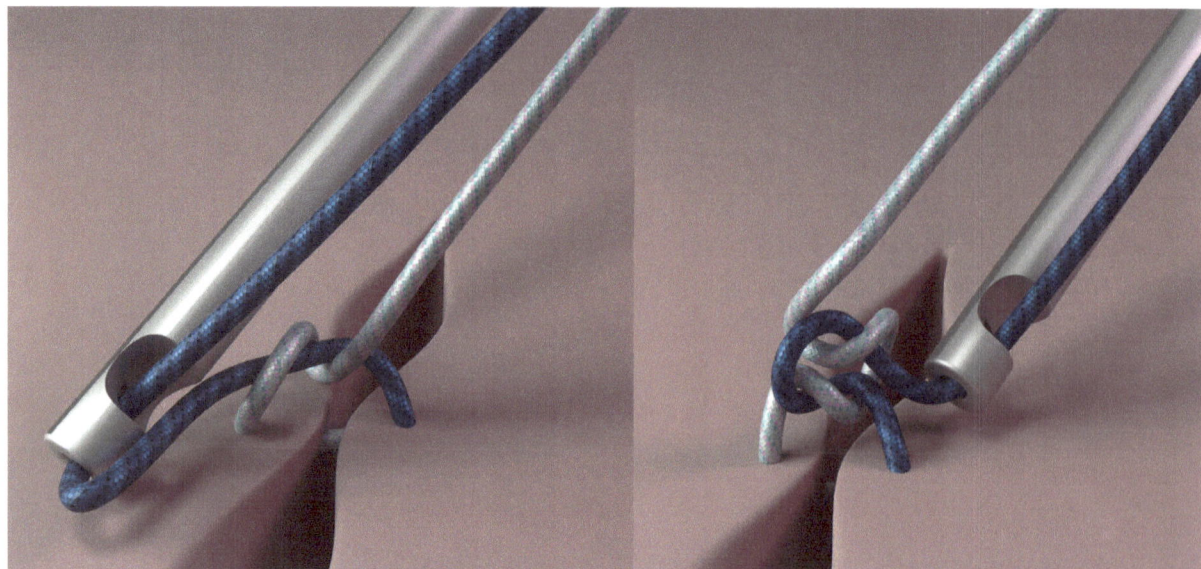

To make knot tying faster, the knot pusher should not be put down between throws. This method maintains an even length of the suture arms but is slower than intracorporeal knot tying [59]. A downside of this approach is that the direction of tension tying down the knot can only be in a line away and towards the trocar. This limitation has made intracorporeal knot tying, rather than extracorporeal, the method of choice for most surgeons.

Pushing technique

Alternatively, the complete knot can be tied, dressed outside the body, and pushed down using a closed knot pusher. Extracorporeal knots can be placed as a noose, semi-locking, or locking flip knots. The knot must be pulled snug outside the body by pulling the ends of the loop apart and pulling on the short end of the suture. The knot is then pushed down as a compact knot. If the knot is not compact before pushing it down, it will be very difficult to tighten it within the body.

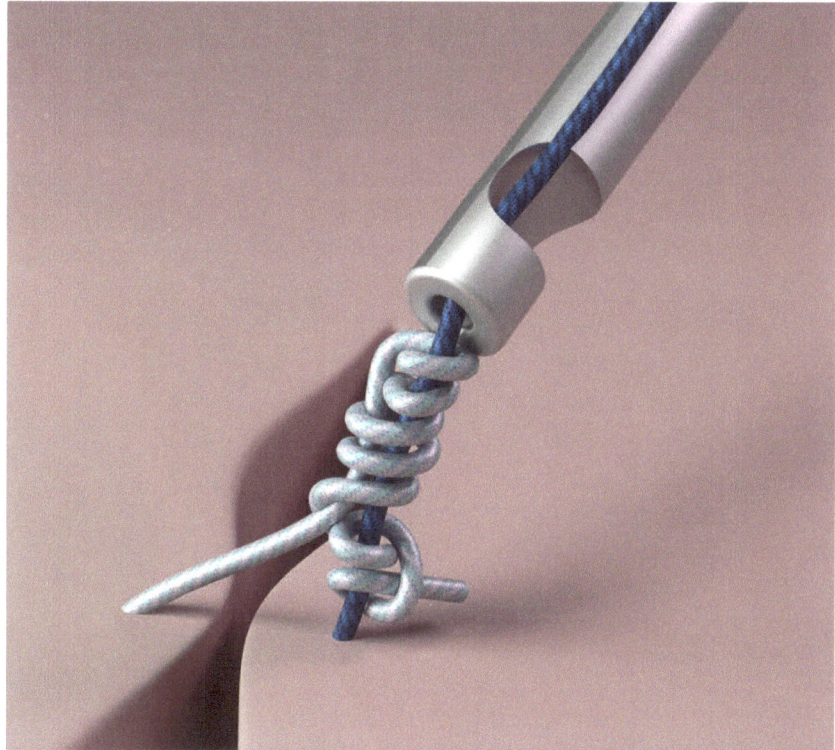

Compared with stacked Overhand knots individually pushed down with a knot pusher, this method is faster, easier, and similar to the pre-made Ethicon Endoloop. It requires using complicated knots that may be unfamiliar to surgeons and requires "dressing" the knot outside the body to ensure that it is compact.

Locking knots have limited applicability outside of arthroscopic surgery. They can be helpful in open surgical procedures where the security of the initial throw is essential, and the ability to pull the suture ends in opposite directions is limited (as in knots tied deep in cavities or with limited space). Even when additional safety throws are used to assure knot security, locking knots are lower profile (less bulky), which minimizes knot extrusion and bulky scar tissue.

Ethicon Endoloop

The Ethicon Endloop is a pretied knot complete with its own disposable plastic knot pusher [60]. The PDS version is likely the most common extracorporeal knot used in laparoscopic surgery and is taught in laparoscopic simulation courses.

The Endoloop is frequently used to tie off the cystic duct or to give extra insurance against bleeding when a larger vessel has been clipped.

As a premade knot, the Endoloop works well, but its security depends upon the proper dressing of the knot by Ethicon's factories. I have not found it as secure as a Melzer knot when hand-tied. It can be rapidly deployed, but since it requires lassoing the tissue end, it cannot tie off a structure that has not already been cut.

For that reason, it has limited use for short structures that can retract, such as a short cystic duct. In cases where a blood vessel or tubular structure must be tied before being cut, it is better to pass a suture around the structure and tie a Melzer or Modified Ethicon knot by hand.

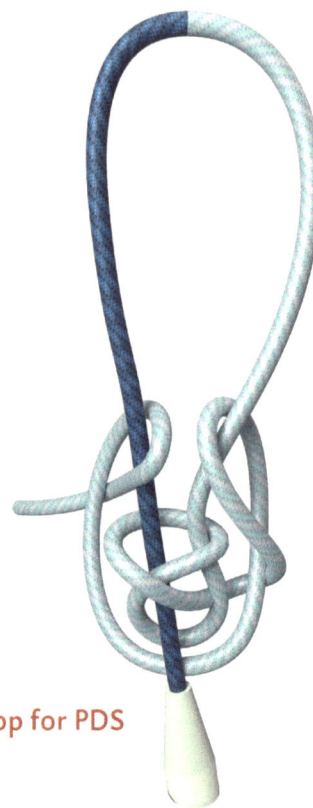

Endoloop for PDS

Semi-locking knots

Extracorporeal semi-locking knots are secure when tissue is not under significant tension, such as when one ligates a cystic duct. However, if the tissue is under tension, the knot should be made secure by at least three half hitches, alternating tension on the two ends.

Melzer knot

The Melzer knot is the most commonly used surgeon-tied extracorporeal knot for PDS suture. It can be tied without first dividing tissue, unlike the preformed Ethicon Endoloop.

Step 1: Tie a double throw knot, the same as the first throw of a Surgeon's knot, and pull on the long end to turn it into a noose.

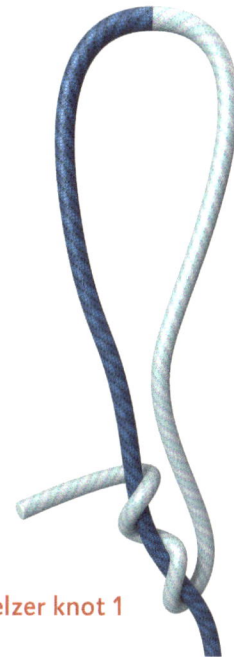

Melzer knot 1

Step 2: Wrap the short end of the suture three times around the loop.

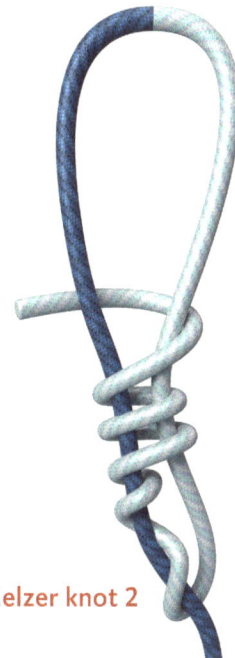

Melzer knot 2

Step 3: Add a half hitch around the post side of the loop.

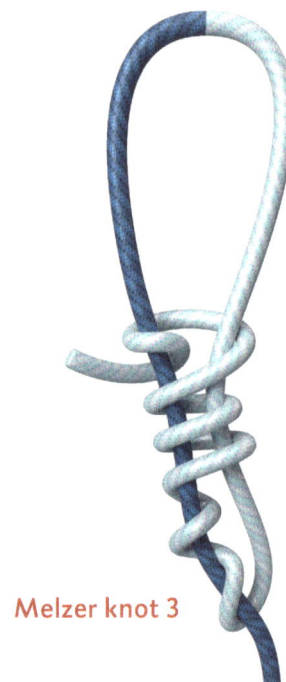

Melzer knot 3

Step 4: Add a second half hitch as a cow hitch.

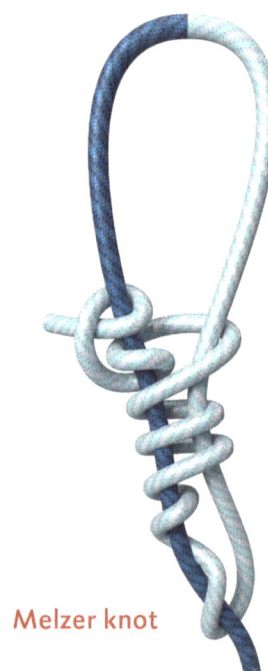

Melzer knot

Tying a Melzer knot

A Melzer knot has the benefits of an Ethicon Endoloop, in that it slides down but is resistant to back slipping. Unlike the Endoloop, it can be tied around a blood vessel before the vessel is cut. The initial steps for tying a Melzer knot are the same as tying a Surgeon's or Nicky knot.

Step 1: Using your right hand and keeping your left palm up, bring the long end of the suture across the palm of your left hand. Grasp the suture between your left thumb and index finger, away from your other fingers.

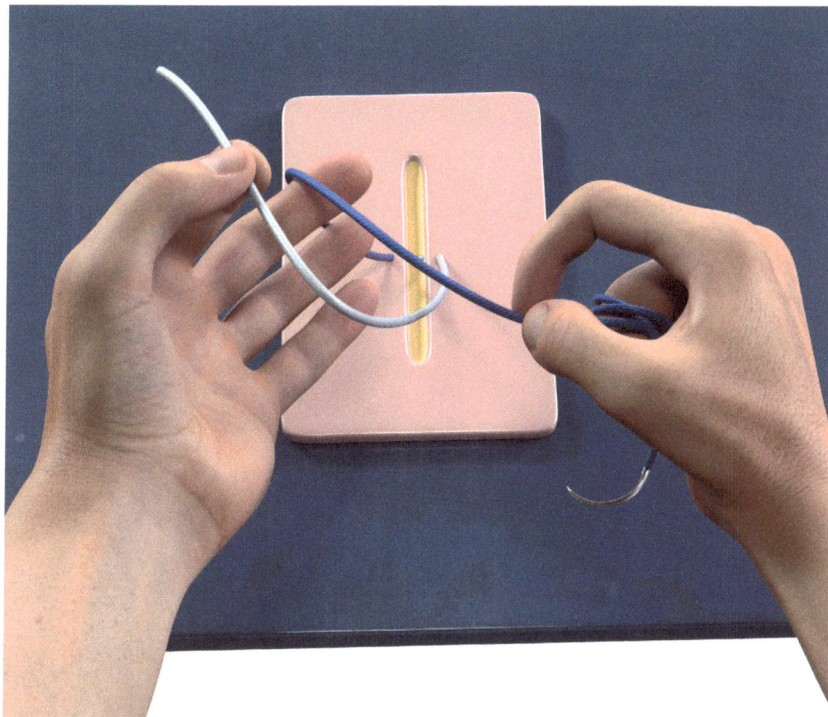

Step 2: Bend your left middle finger under the short end of the suture. Prepare to catch the short end of the suture between the back of your left middle finger and front of your left ring finger.

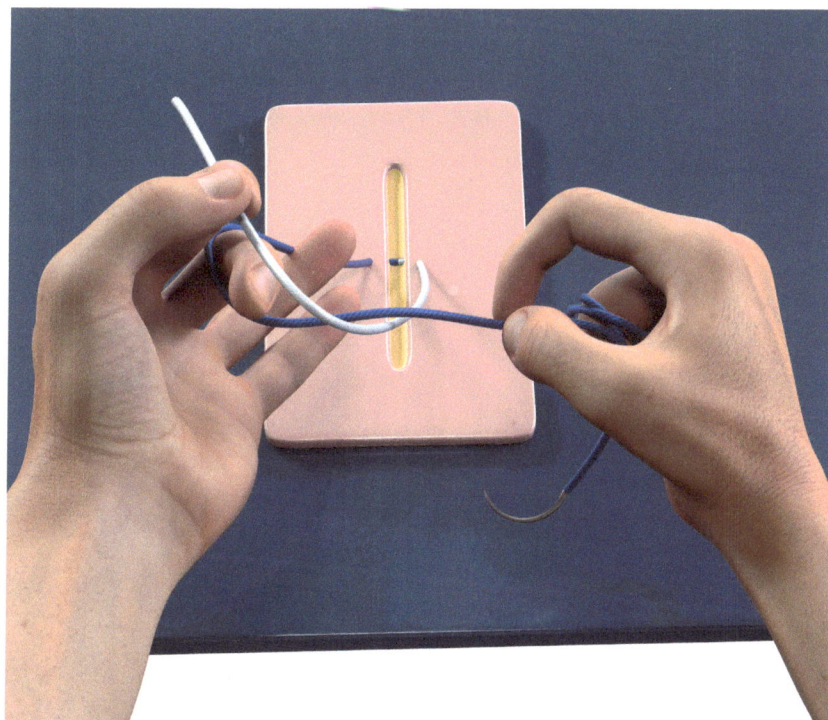

Step 3: Catch the short end of the suture between your left middle and ring fingers. Release the grip on the suture between your thumb and index finger.

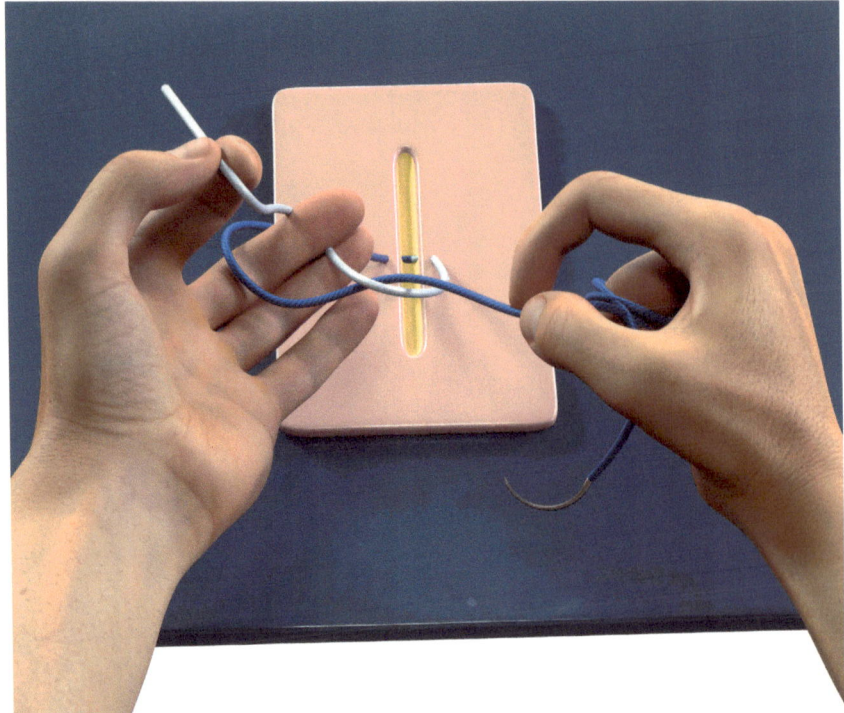

Step 4: Pull the tip of the short end of the suture under the long end.

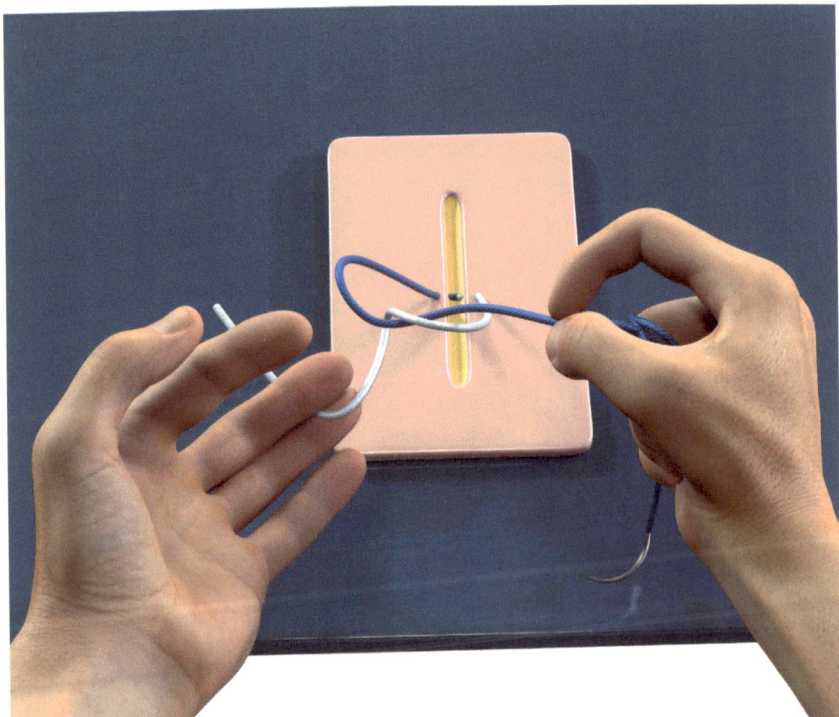

Step 5: Place your left hand back under the loop formed by the suture, keeping your palm face up. Grasp the short end of the suture between your right middle and ring fingers.

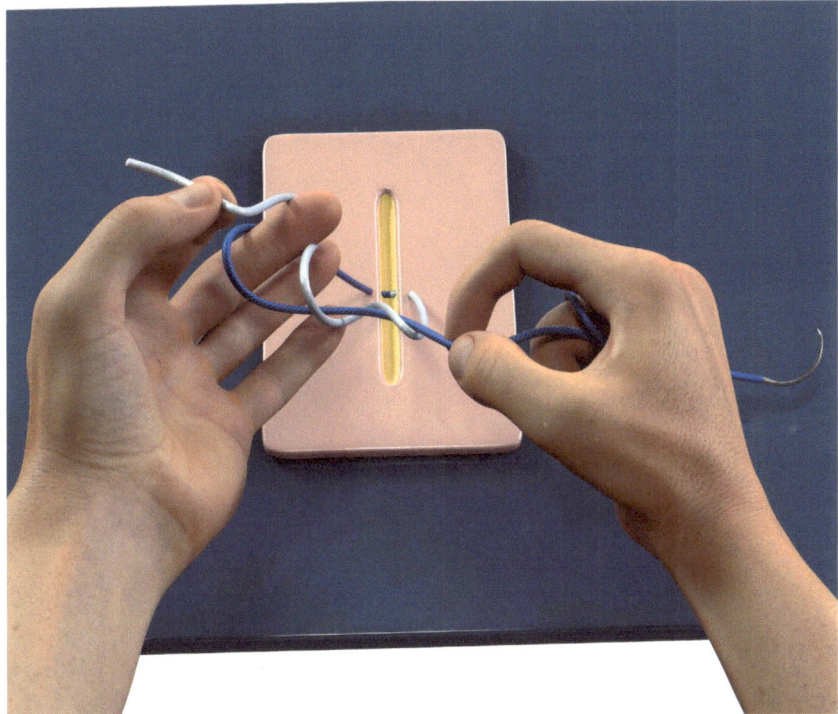

Step 6: Pull up on the suture with your right hand to form a post. Pull up with your left hand to tighten the short end of the suture around the post, dressing the knot.

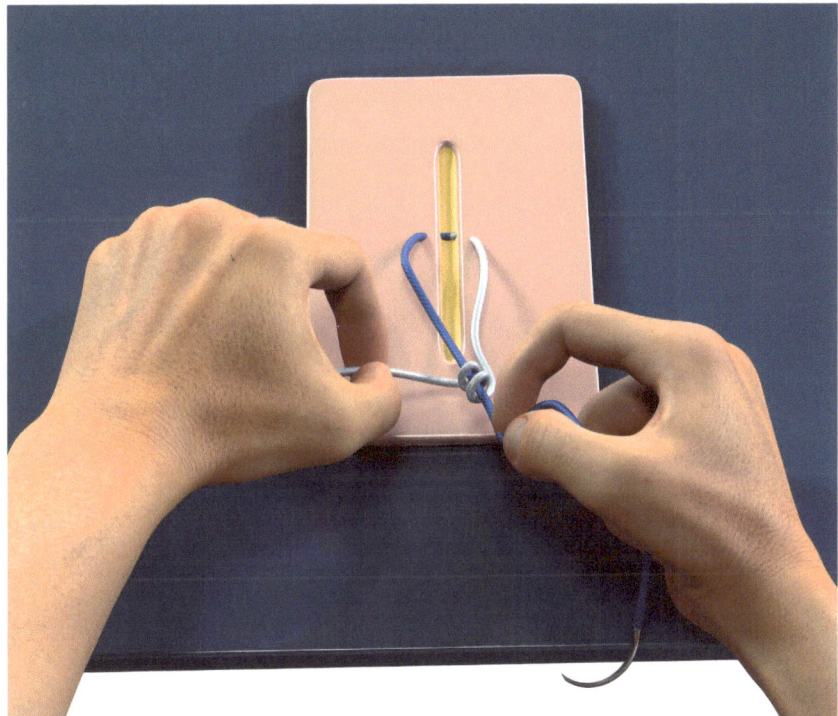

Step 7: Using your left hand, wrap the suture three times around both limbs of the loop formed through the tissue. You can keep these wraps from loosening by holding the end of the suture between your right middle and ring fingers when passing the end around with your left hand.

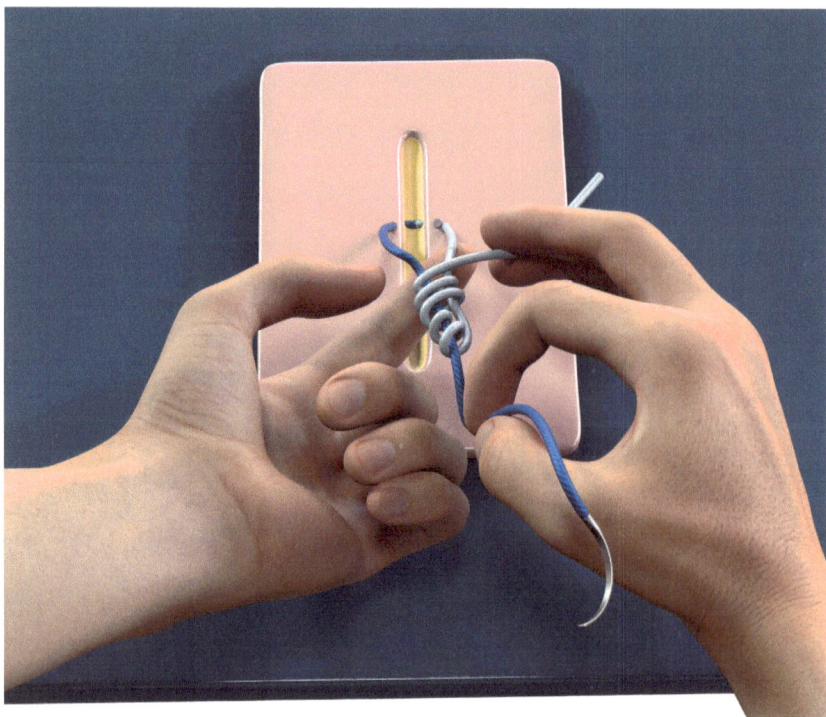

Step 8: Using your left hand, add a half hitch around the post.

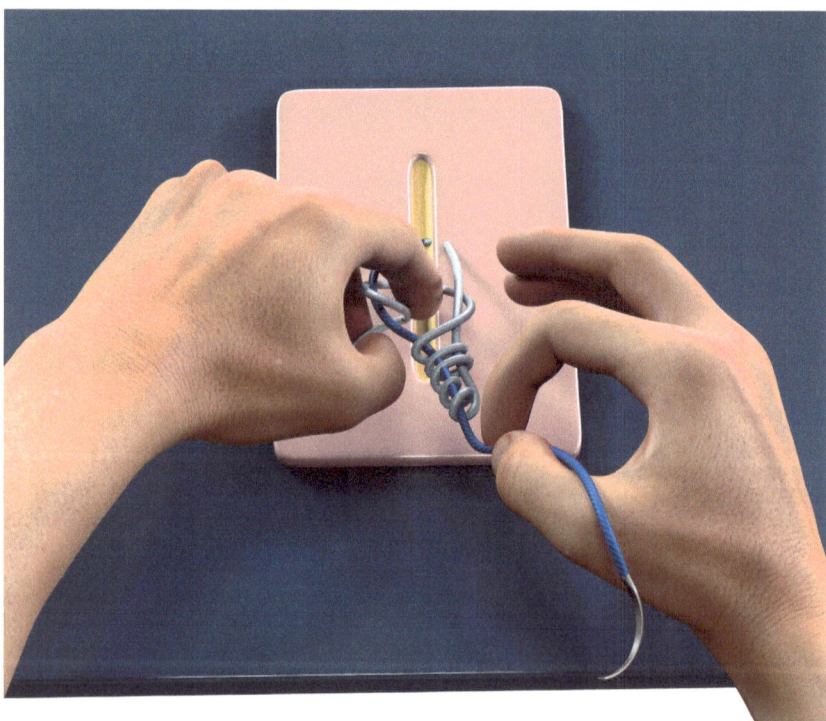

Step 9: Add a second half hitch around the post end of the suture and tighten the knot in place. To dress the knot, put your left hand under the loop that goes through the tissue and pull upwards to tighten the knot. This assures that it will not slip back after it is slid down. Finally, slide the knot down with your hands or a pusher.

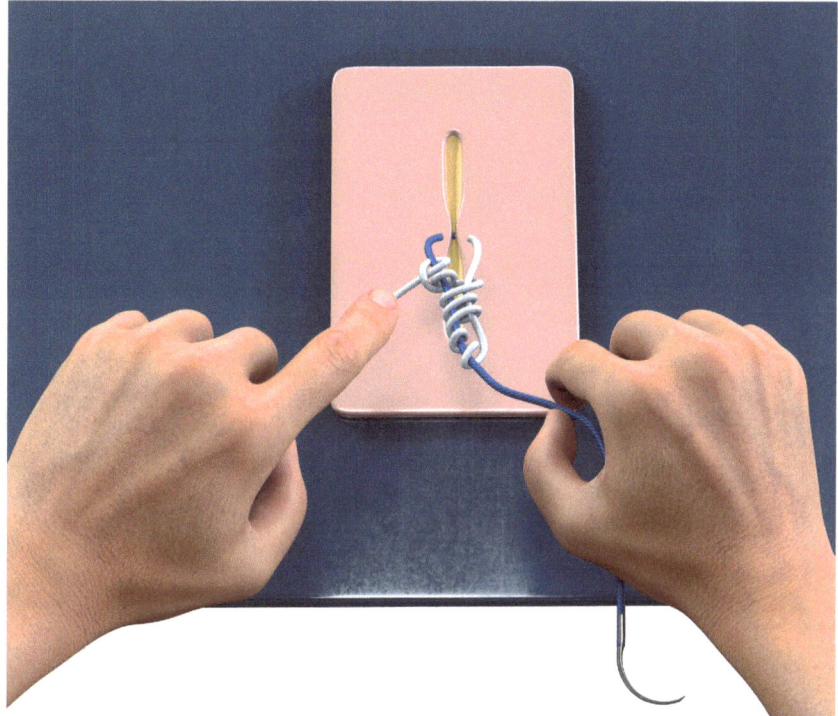

Video of tying Melzer knot:
https://www.youtube.com/watch?v=I9bGO2BnX7k

Semilocking knot summary

Alternatives to the Melzer knot are the Savoi Roeder [61] and Modified Ethicon Sliding knot [60]. Both slide down easily with monofilament sutures yet resist loosening in response to tissue tension.

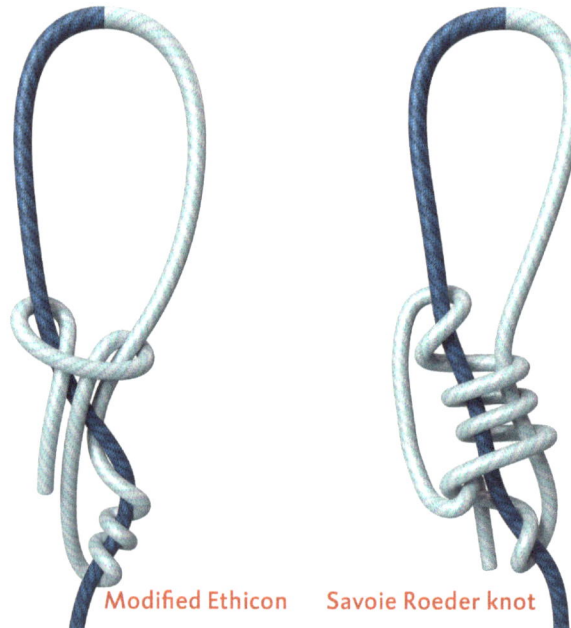

Modified Ethicon   Savoie Roeder knot

All semi-locking knots function similarly to a nylon cable tie and resist back slippage. Technically, ratcheting knots do not exist [62]. Functionally, as they are tied down, specific knots change the angle of the strands of suture at the bottom of the knot. The forces switch from an up/down direction to a side-to-side direction, which reduces their tendency to slip. With the Modified Ethicon Knot, additional wraps can be placed proximally for added security.

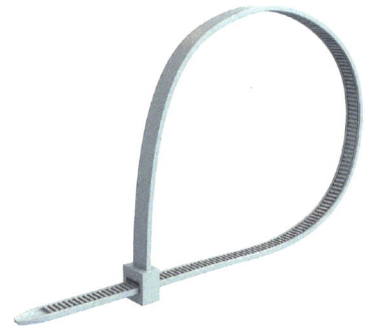

Locking knots

Locking knots are seldom used in general or laparoscopic surgery but are common in arthroscopic surgery. They have an advantage over semi-locking knots in that the knot flips into a locked position if the non-post end is pulled upwards, reducing the chance of accidentally slipping backward. In practice, the flipping of the knot results in some loosening of the loop, and locking knots have been shown to lack security unless additional half hitches are added [40, 41, 61]. There is considerable variability even among experienced surgeons in the security of locking knots [63].

SMC knot

The Samsung Medical Center knot [39, 41] is considered superior to a sliding knot because it can be locked by pulling on the short end after it is slipped down. In practice, this results in some loop widening with poorer tissue apposition. The locking property of the knot itself is not secure unless three reversing half hitches on alternating posts are added [45].

Step 1: The post (blue) side should be half the length of the sliding (cyan) limb. Pass the end of the suture over the post, then wrap behind the post and over both parts of the loop.

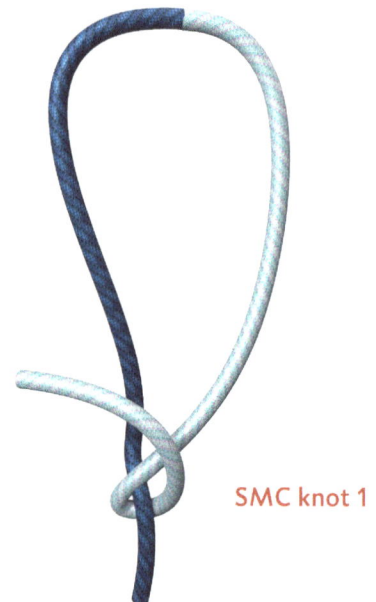

SMC knot 1

Step 2: Wrap the end of the suture around the post part within the loop.

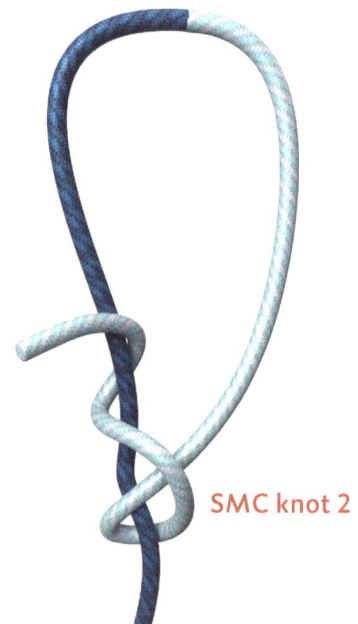

SMC knot 2

Step 3: Bring the end of the suture out between the sliding and post parts of the knot.

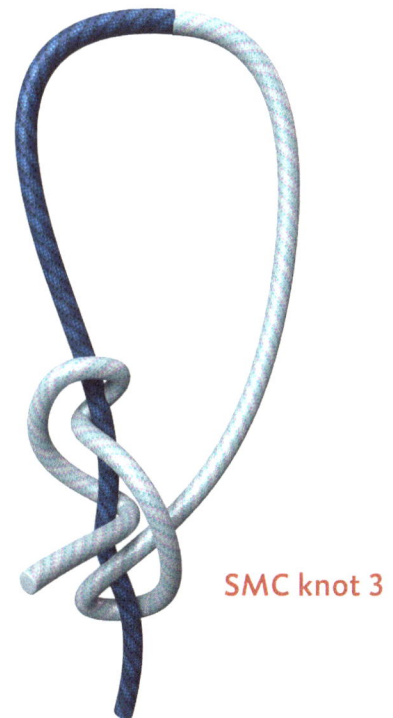

SMC knot 3

Step 4: After sliding the knot down, pull up on the end of the suture to lock the knot.

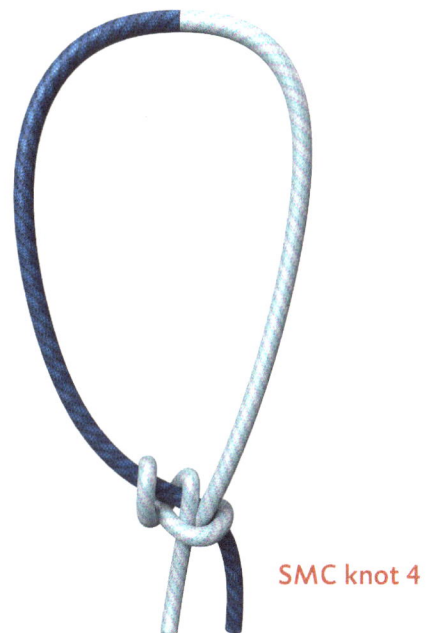

SMC knot 4

Tying a SMC knot

The SMC knot is tied mostly with your left hand, while holding a crossed loop of suture in your right hand.

Step 1: Hold the long end of the suture with your right hand and the short end with your left hand, without crossing the two ends.

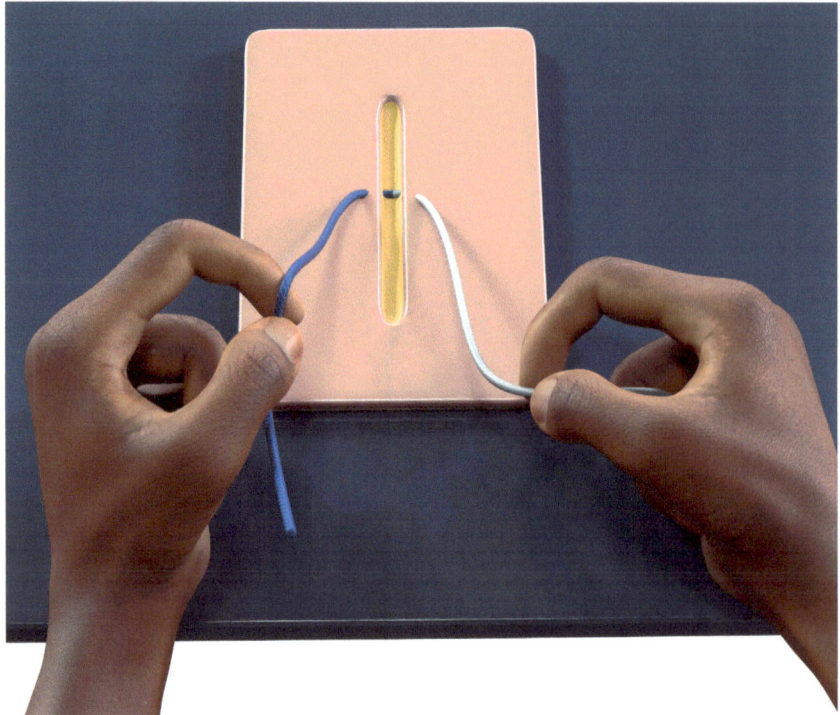

Step 2: Turn your left hand upwards and use your right hand to cross the short end over the long end. Pinch these two sutures together with your left index finger and thumb.

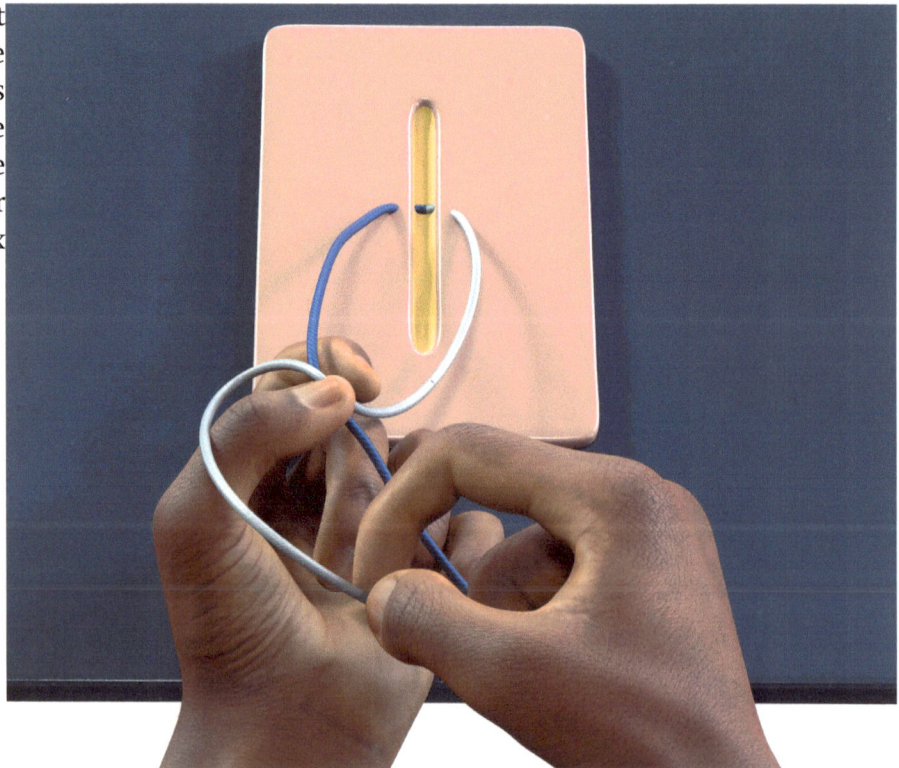

Step 3: With your right hand, move the short end of the suture behind the loop held in your left hand.

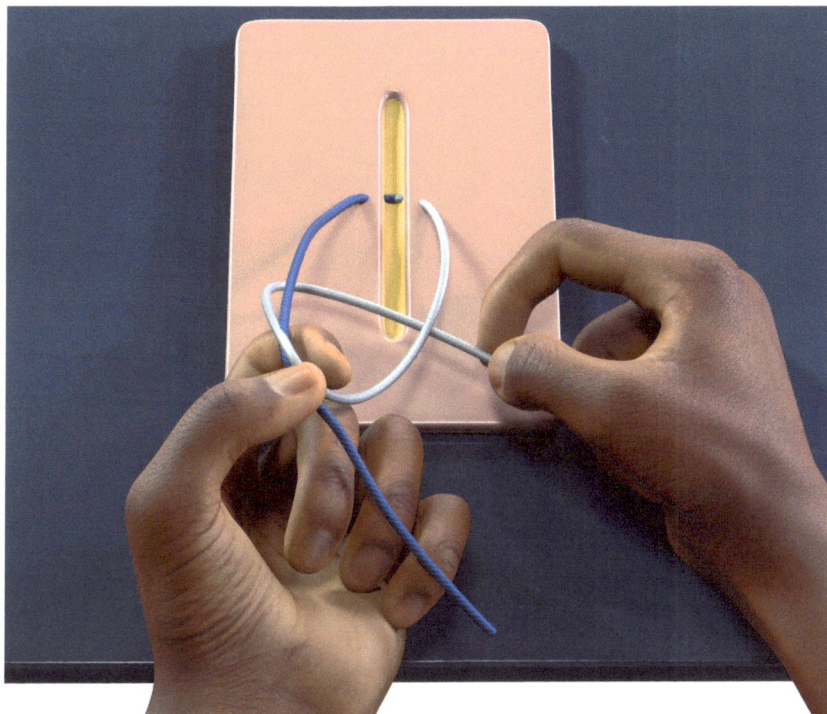

Step 4: Again, with your right hand, wrap the short end around the loop held in your left hand.

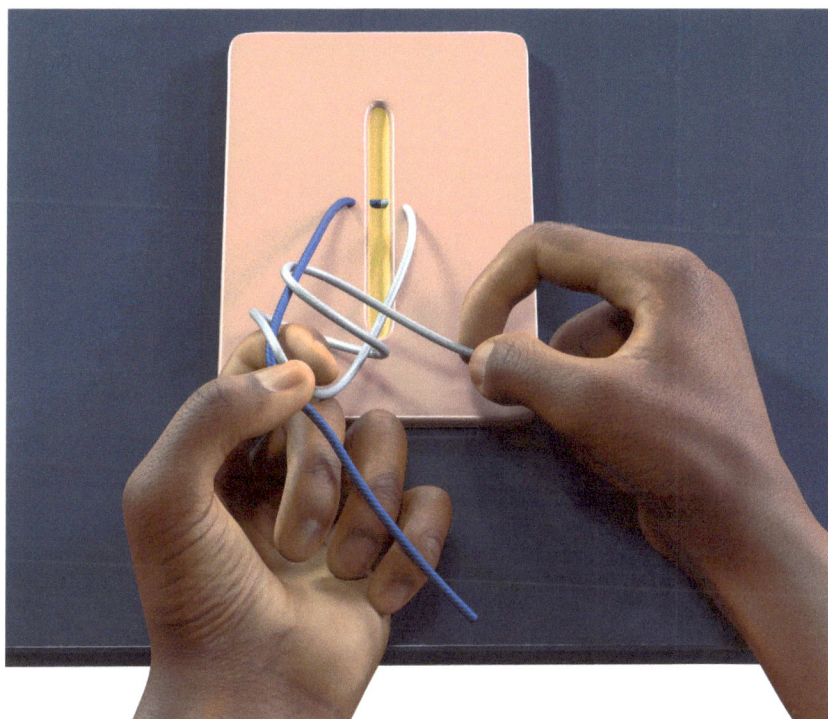

Step 5: Loop the short end just around the long end of the suture closest to the tissue.

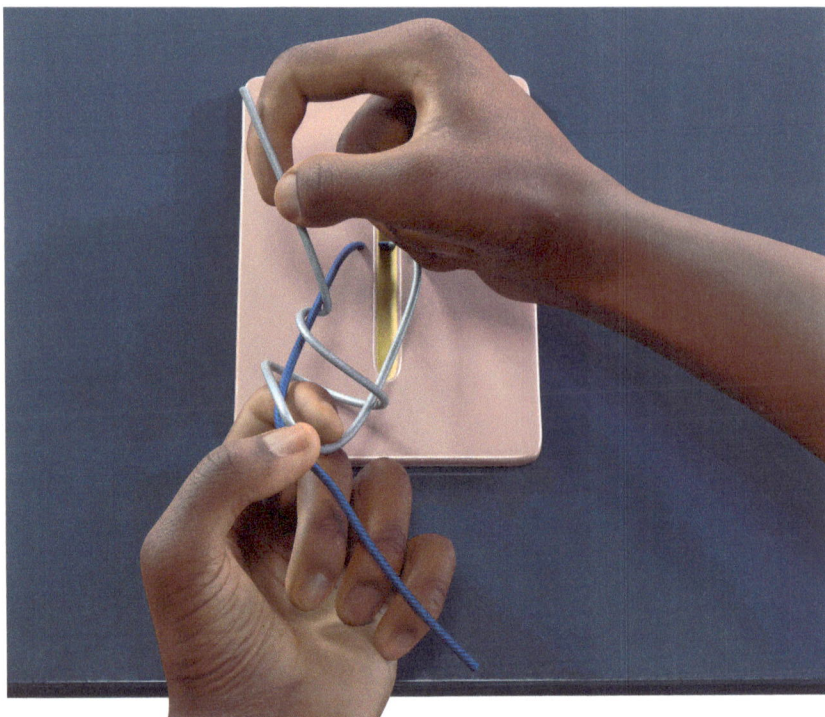

Step 6: Bring the short end of the suture under and up around the long end of the suture closest to your left hand.

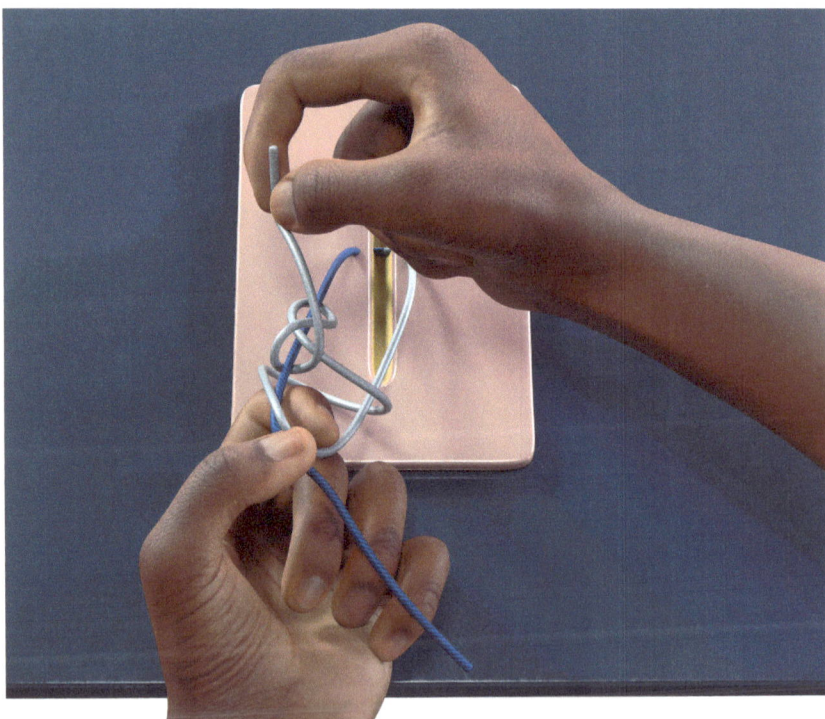

Step 7: Pull up on the long end of the suture to slide the knot into place. After that is done, pull up on the short end to lock the knot.

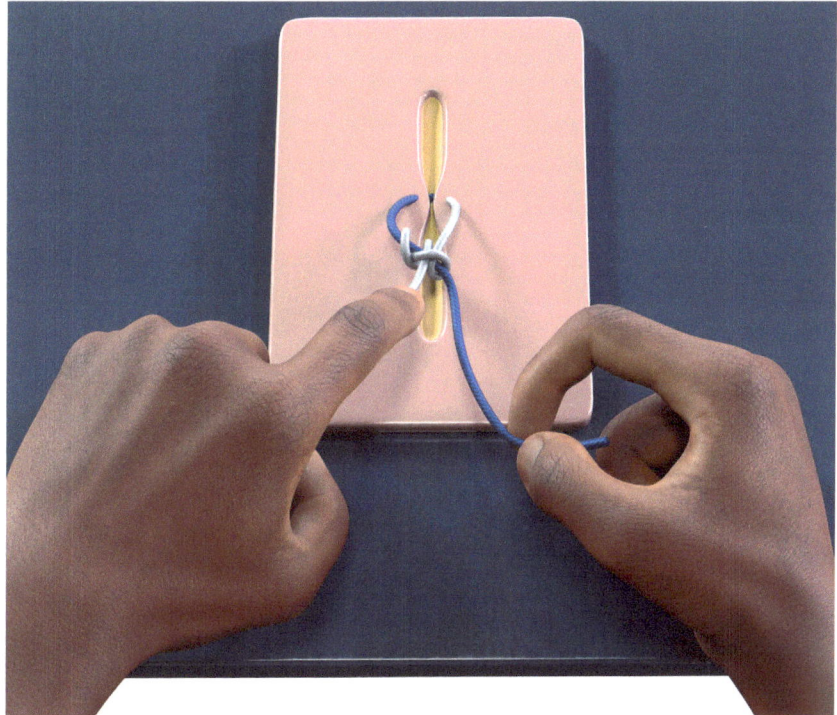

Dines Slider

Like the SMC knot, the Dines Slider [39, 64] can be slipped down and flipped to lock in place. Compared to the SMC knot, it is less apt to slip [65]. Like the SMC knot, flipping the knot to lock the suture results in some widening of the loop - a flaw in all locking extracorporeal knots [40]. Some studies have shown that, like other locking extracorporeal knots, additional reversed half hitches are required to assure knot security [67].

Step 1: The post (blue) side should be half the length of the sliding (cyan) limb. Make a bend in the sliding end over the post side.

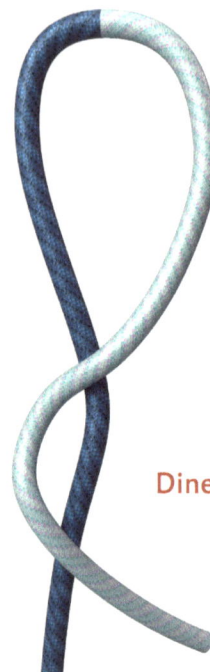

Dines knot 1

Step 2: Bring the suture under the post side and up through the small loop formed in step 1, then down through the large loop.

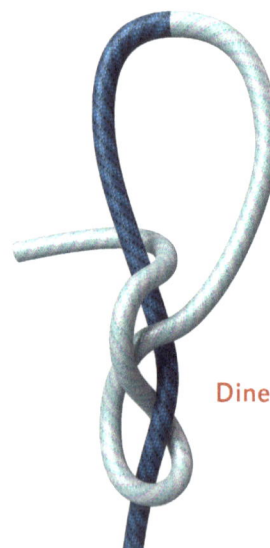

Dines knot 2

Step 3: Bring the suture around the post side of the large loop and pass it under the post in the small loop formed in step 1.

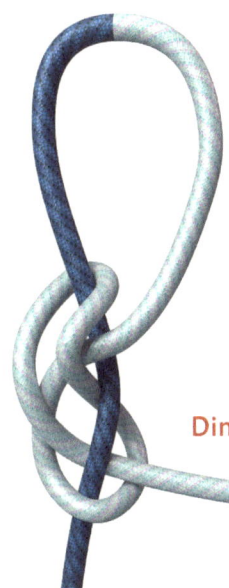

Dines knot 3

Tying a Dines Slider knot

The following steps are to tie a Dines Slider

Step 1: Cross a loop of the short end of the suture across the long end and pinch the two sutures together with your left thumb and index fingers.

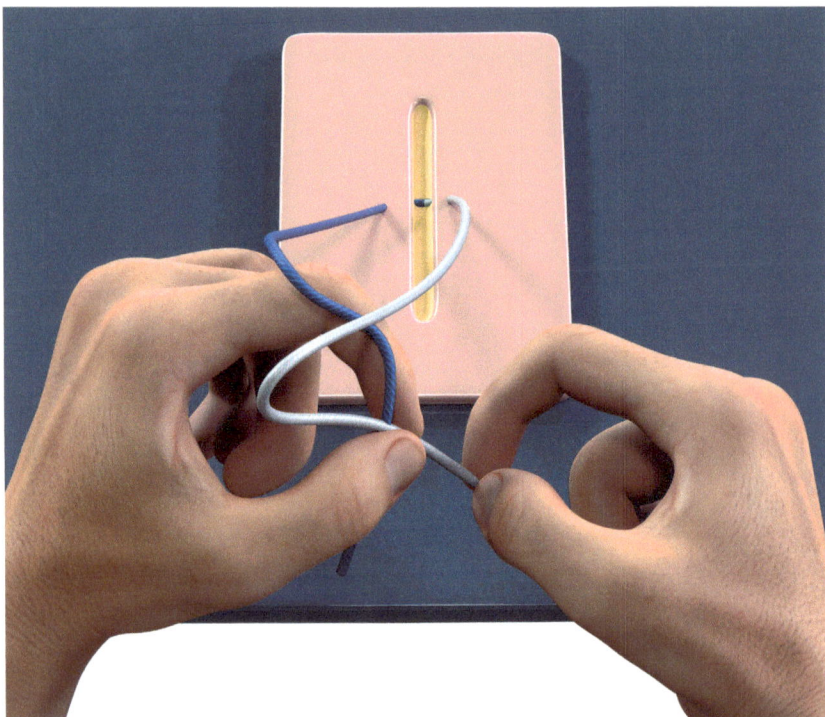

Step 2: Pull the short end up through the space between the short and long end of the sutures with your right hand.

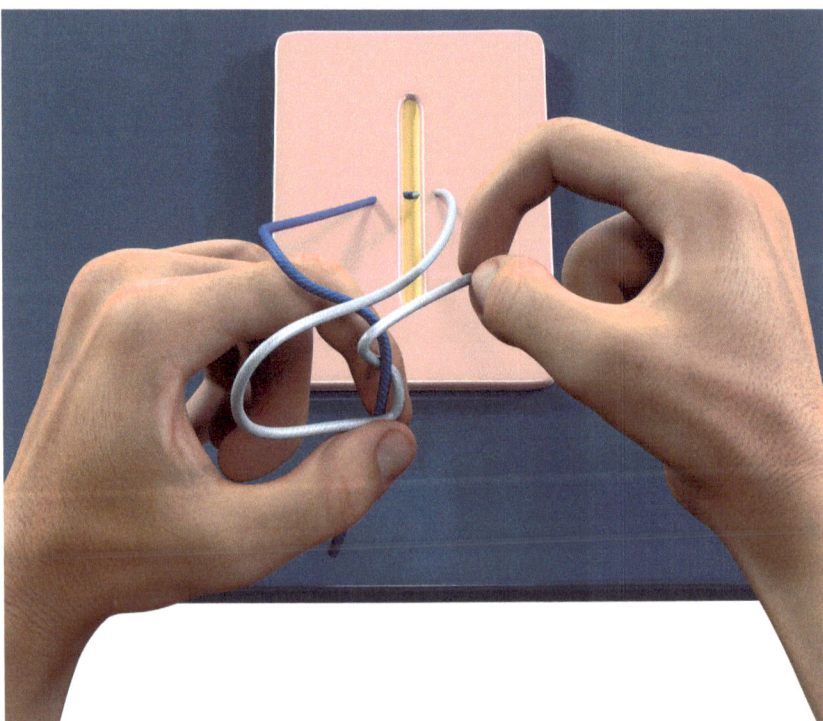

Step 3: Pass the short end of the suture around the long end closest to the tissue.

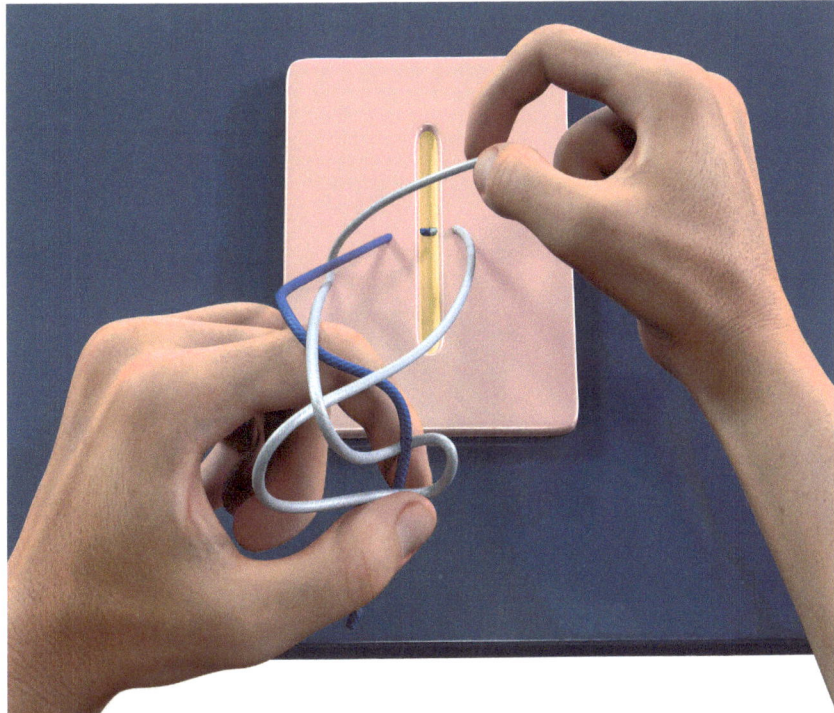

Step 4: Pass the short end under the long end of the suture close to where the two sutures are held by your left hand.

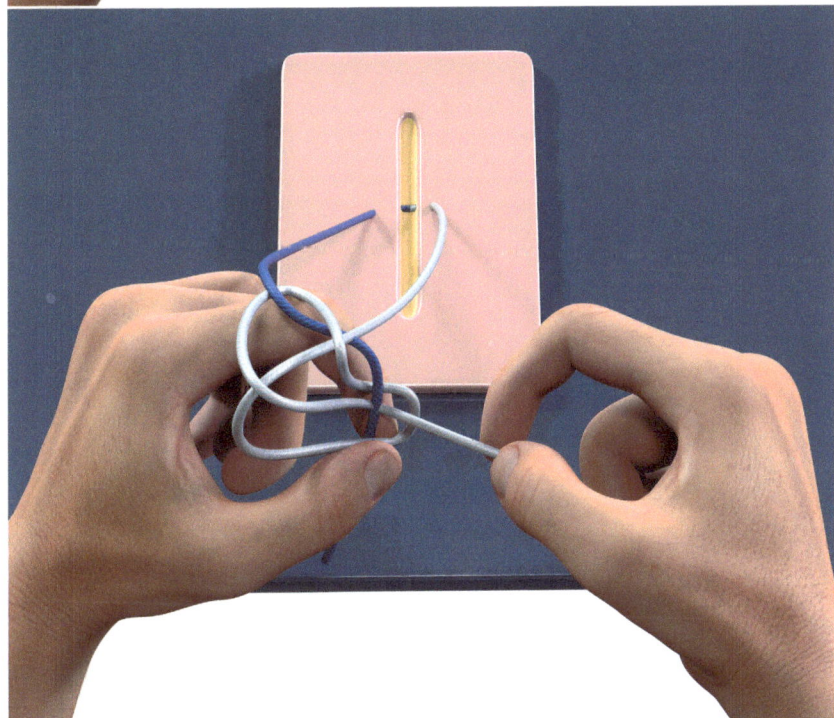

Step 5: Sliding the knot down and then pull up on the short end to lock the knot.

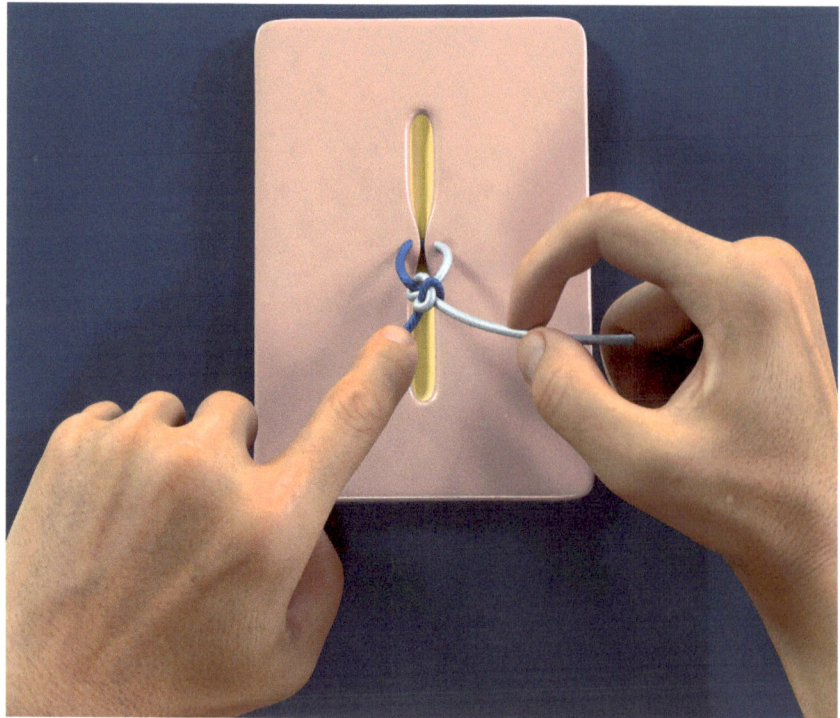

Outback knot

The Outback knot has somewhat less widening of the loop when locked down compared with the SMC and Dines slider and may be more secure [43].

Step 1: The post (blue) side should be half the length of the sliding (cyan) limb. Tie a half hitch with the sliding end under and then over the post limb.

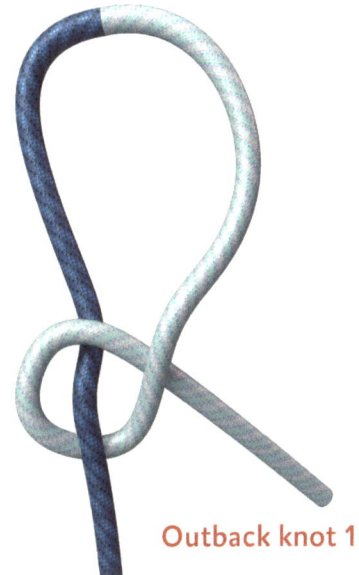

Outback knot 1

Step 2: Flip the loop in the sliding limb over the post limb.

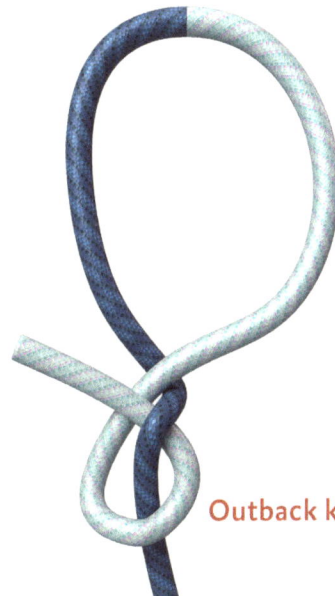

Outback knot 2

Step 3: Pass the end of the suture down through the big loop.

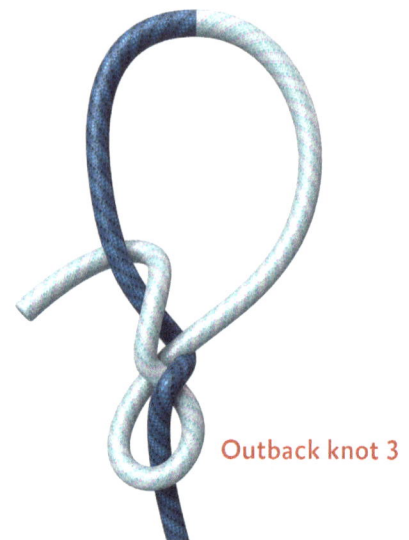

Outback knot 3

Step 4: Pass the end of the suture through the small loop formed in step 1. Slide the knot down.

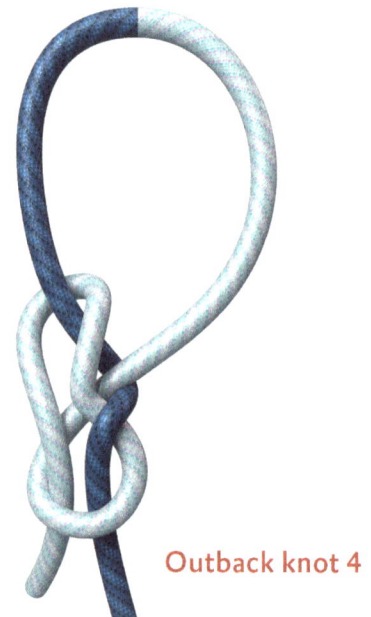

Outback knot 4

Step 5: Pull up on the end of the suture to lock the knot.

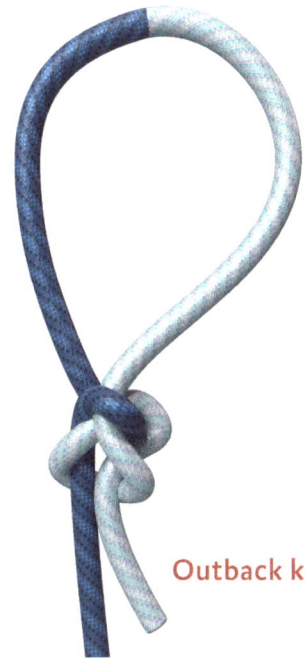

Outback knot 5

Tying an Outback knot

An Outback knot can be tied, slipped down, and then locked into place. It is seldom used in general surgery but is one of the simplest and most reliable knots in arthroscopic surgery where a locking knot is desired.

Step 1: With your right palm face down, wrap the long end of the suture around the middle part of your right middle finger. Hold the short end of the suture with your left hand. Make sure the long end of the suture is farther away from you than the short end held by your right hand. Curl your right index finger under both the short and long ends of the suture.

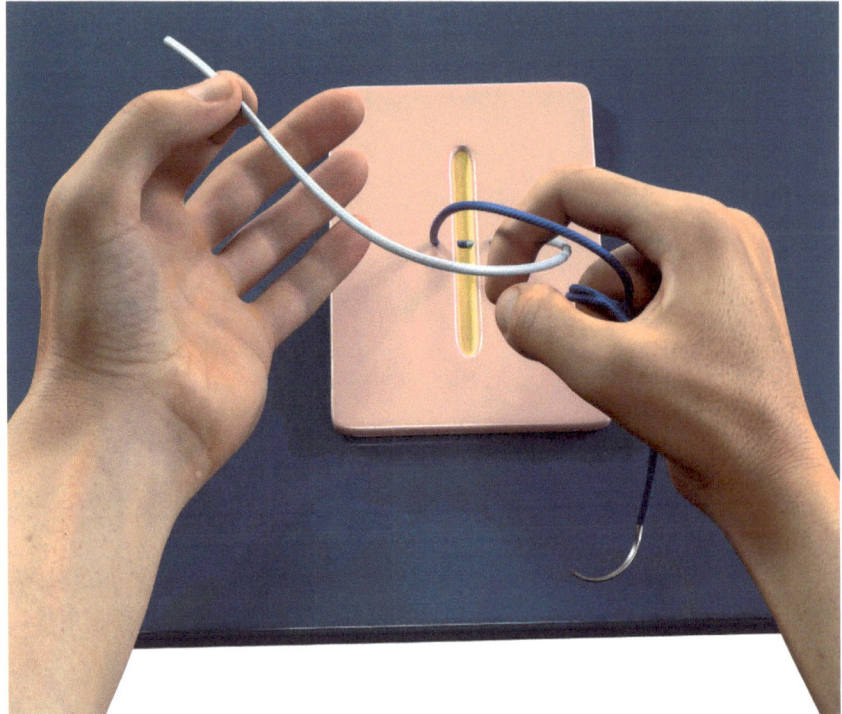

Step 2: Bring your right thumb under the loop and grasp the short end between your right thumb and index fingers.

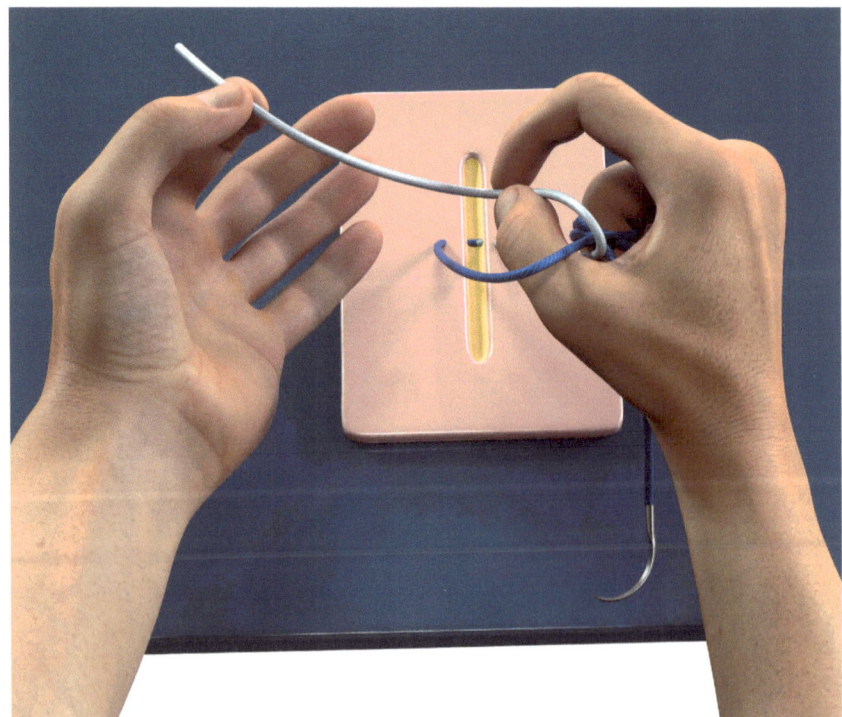

Step 3: Let go of the short end of the suture with your left hand. Pull the short end of the suture under the long end using your right index finger and thumb.

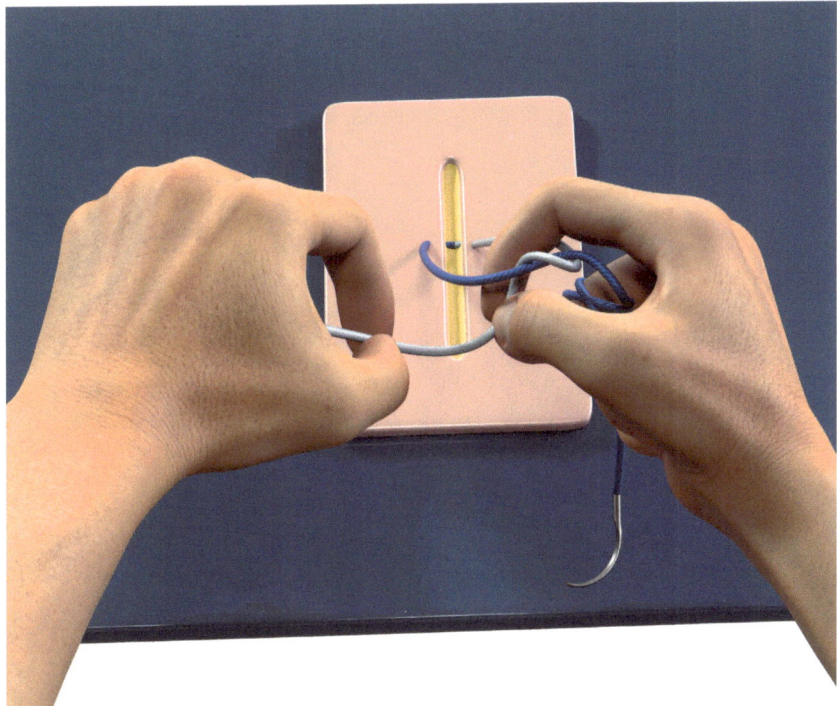

Step 4: Move the short end of the suture to your right, under your right hand, to form a loop.

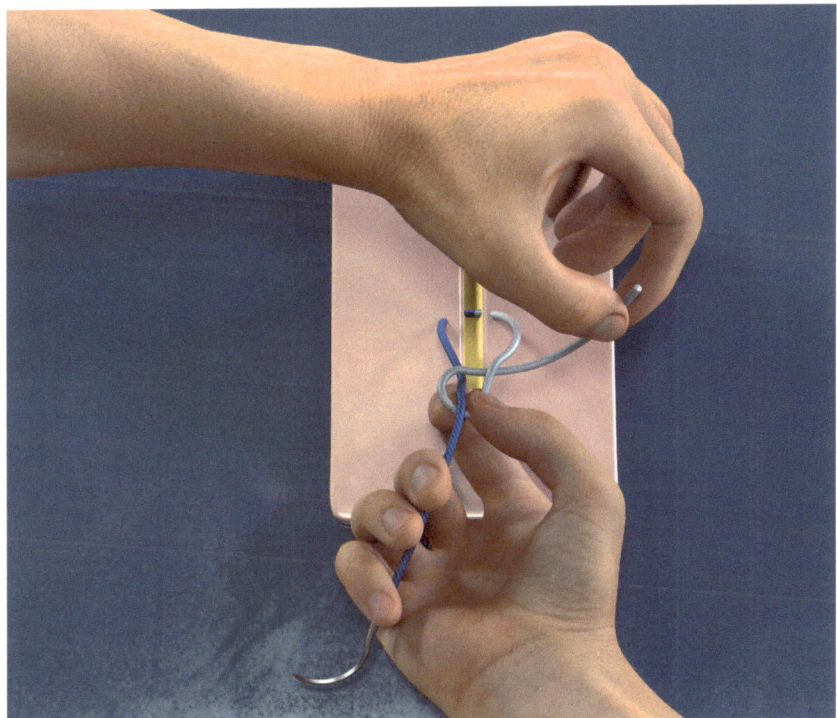

Step 5: Flip the loop over by holding it in your right hand and turning your palm down.

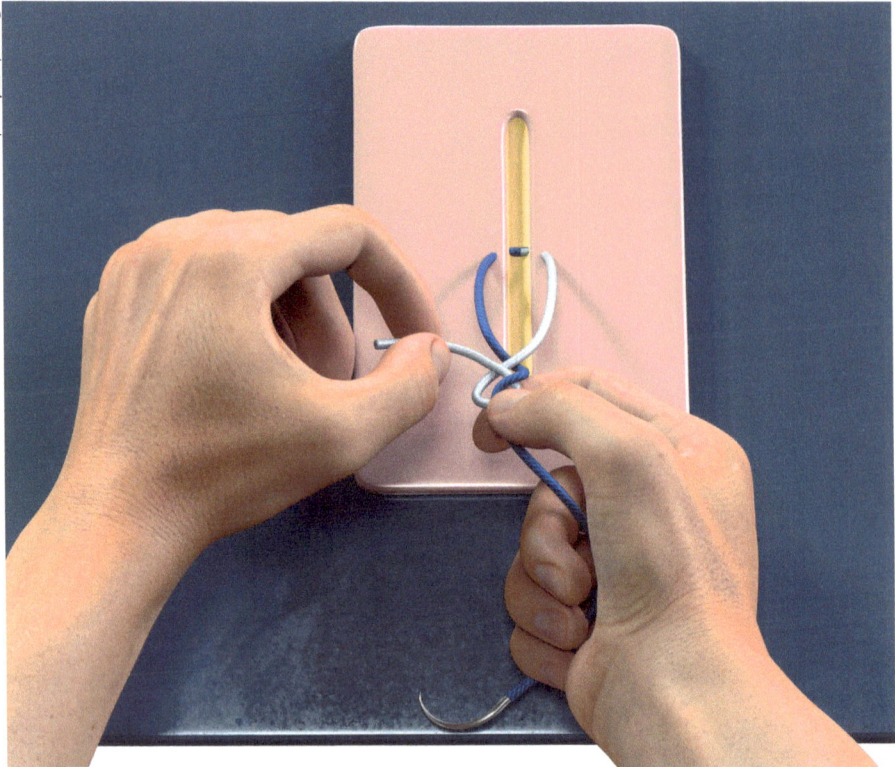

Step 6: Place the short end of the suture down through the loop which goes through the tissue.

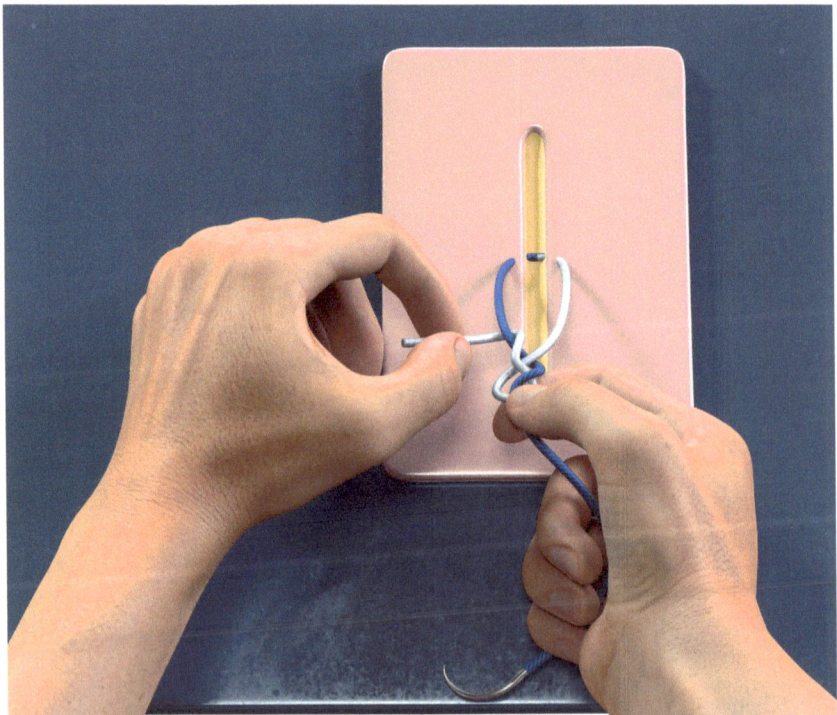

Step 7: Place the short end of the suture down through the loop which is towards you. With your right hand, pull up on the suture to form a post and slide the knot down to appose the tissue.

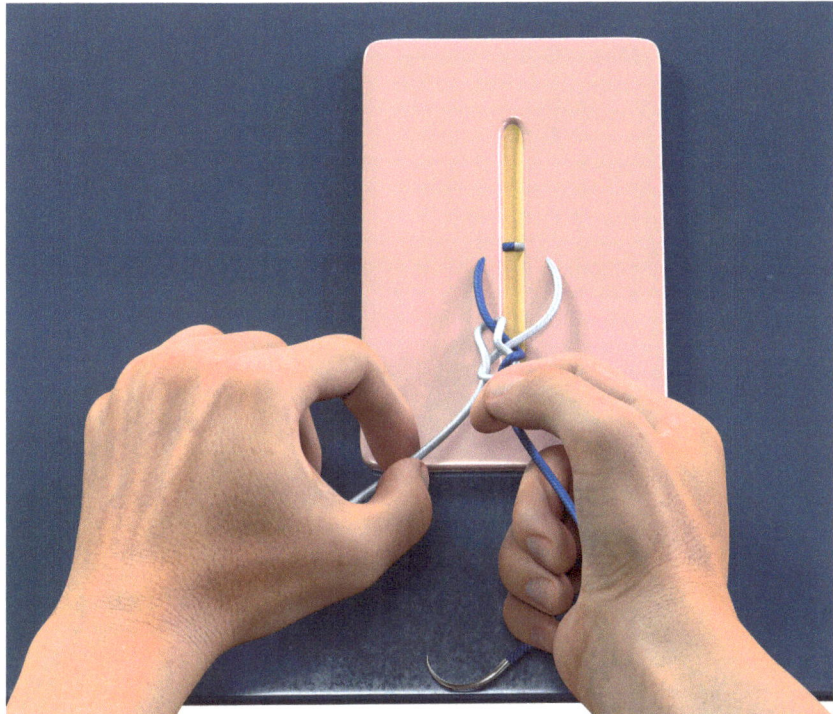

Step 8: Pull up on the short end of the suture in your left hand to lock the knot.

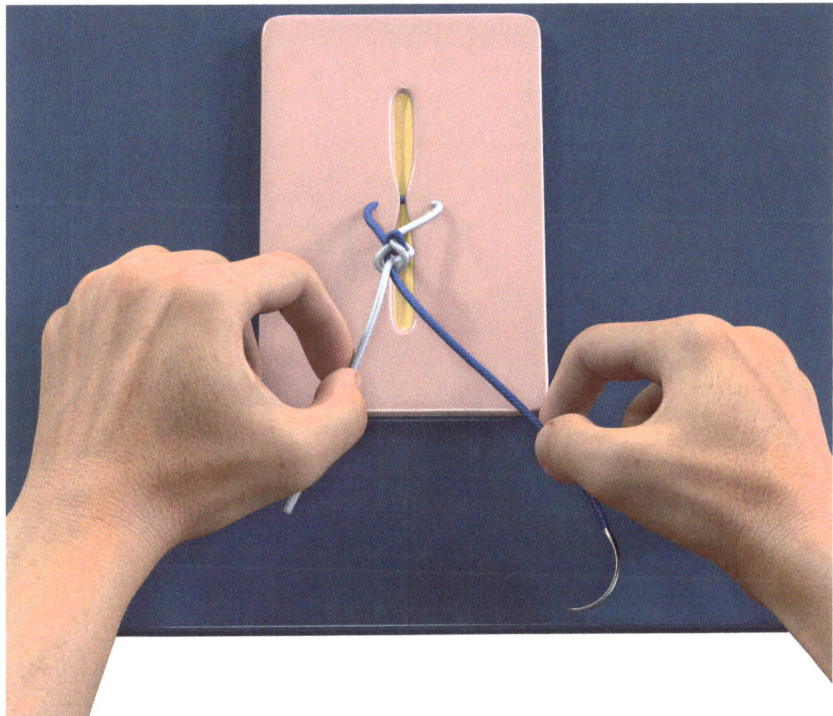

Video of tying Outback knot:
https://vimeo.com/191751818

Gea knot

Surgeons at the Manuel Gea Gonzalez General Hospital in Mexico City developed the Gea Extracorporeal knot and claimed that it is superior to the Roeder knot [68, 69]. Testing it with paracord, I do not find it as secure as the Melzer knot, as the loop widens significantly before the knot locks.

Step 1: Tie a double throw knot (the same as the first throw of a Surgeon's knot) and pull up on the post side to turn it into a noose.

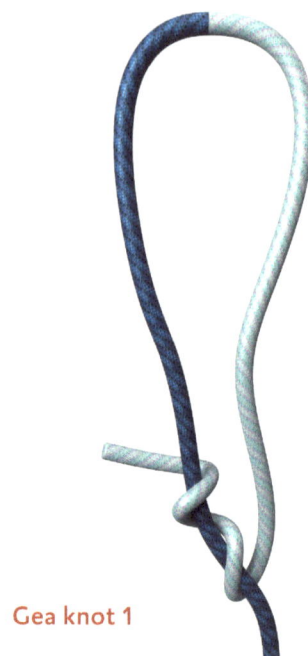

Gea knot 1

Step 2: Wrap the suture once around both sides of the loop.

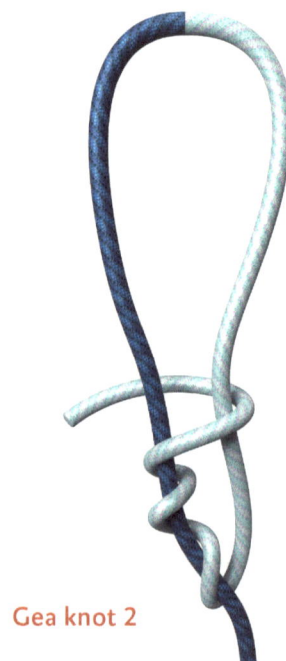

Gea knot 2

Step 3: Add a half hitch around the post limb of the loop.

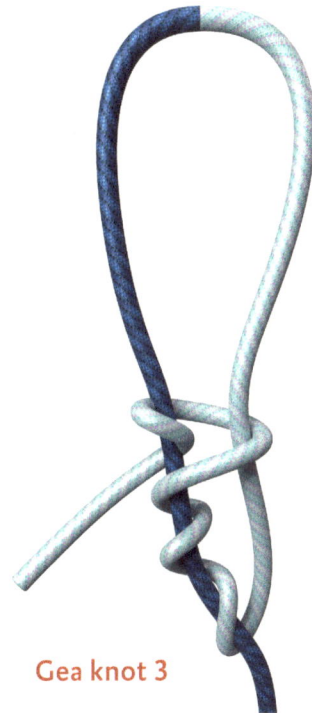

Gea knot 3

Step 4: Run the end of the suture back through the lower part of the knot.

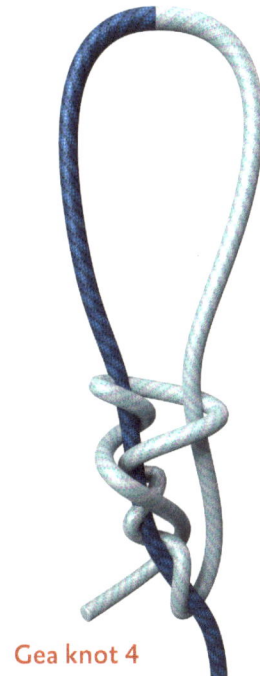

Gea knot 4

Tying a Gea Knot

Step 1: Using your right hand and keeping your left palm up, bring the long end of the suture across the palm of your left hand.

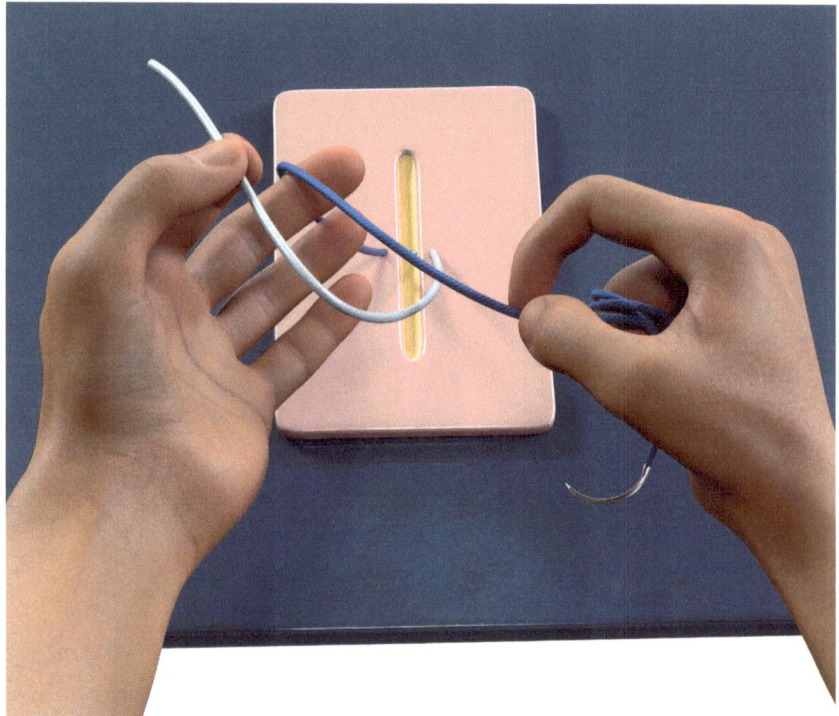

Step 2: Bend your left middle finger under the short end of the suture, preparing to catch the short end of the suture between the back of your left middle finger and front of your left ring finger.

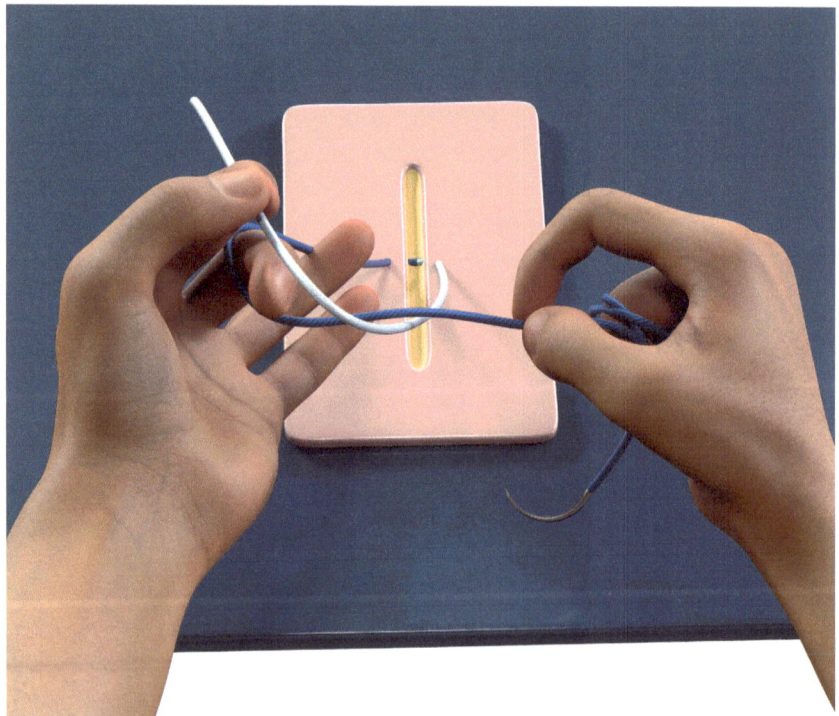

Step 3: Catch the short end of the suture between your left middle and ring finger and release the grip on the suture between your thumb and index finger.

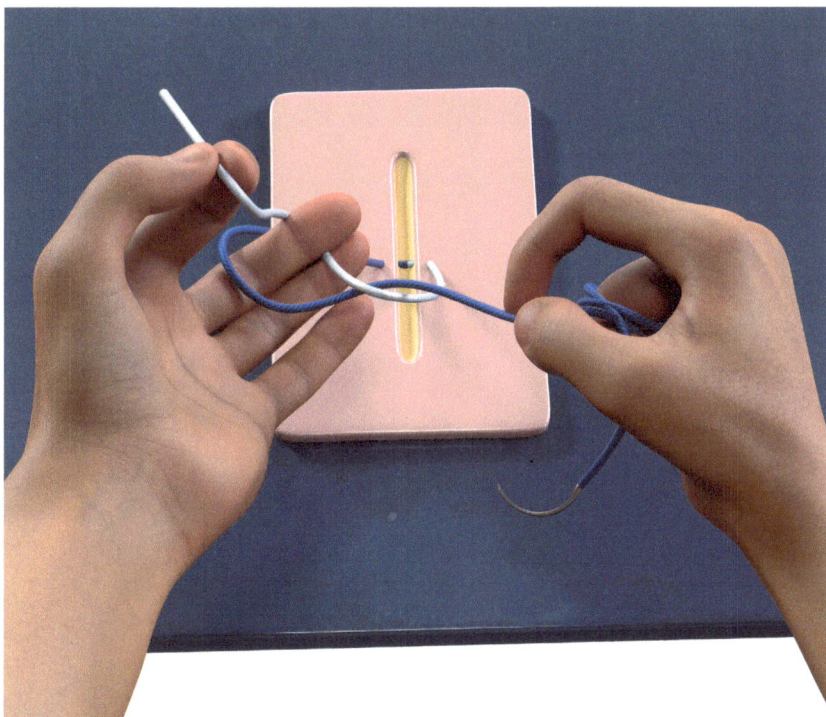

Step 4: Pull the short end of the suture under the long end, so as to form an overhand knot.

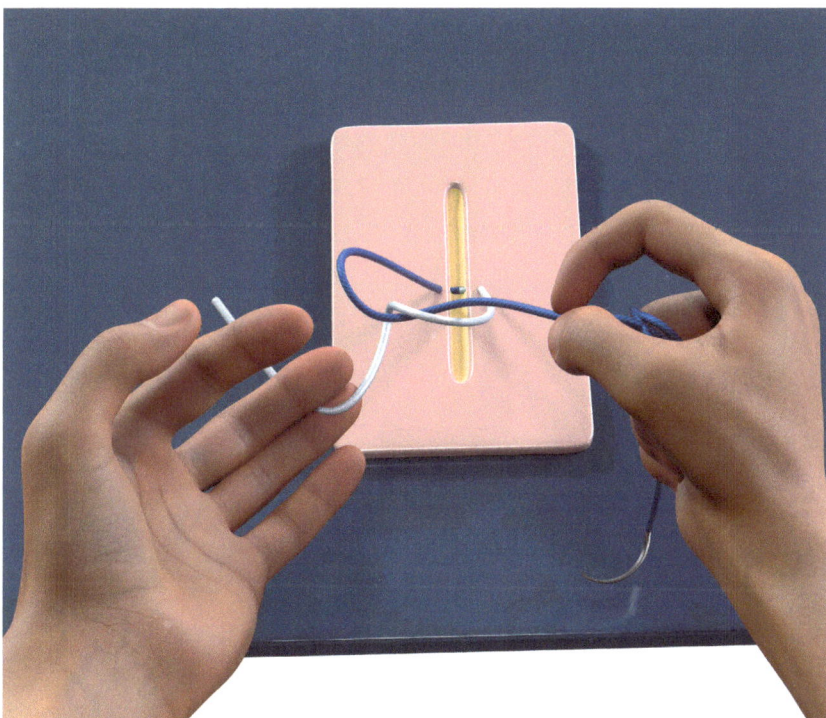

Step 5: Slide your right thumb under the overhand loop and grasp the short end again and pull it through, forming the beginning of a Surgeon's knot.

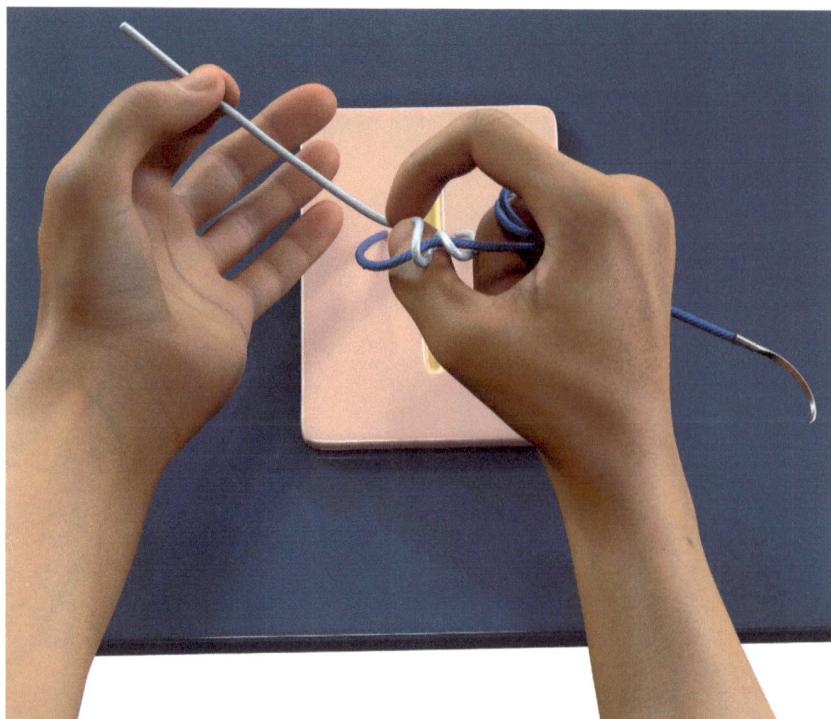

Step 6: Pull up on the long end to convert the knot to a noose.

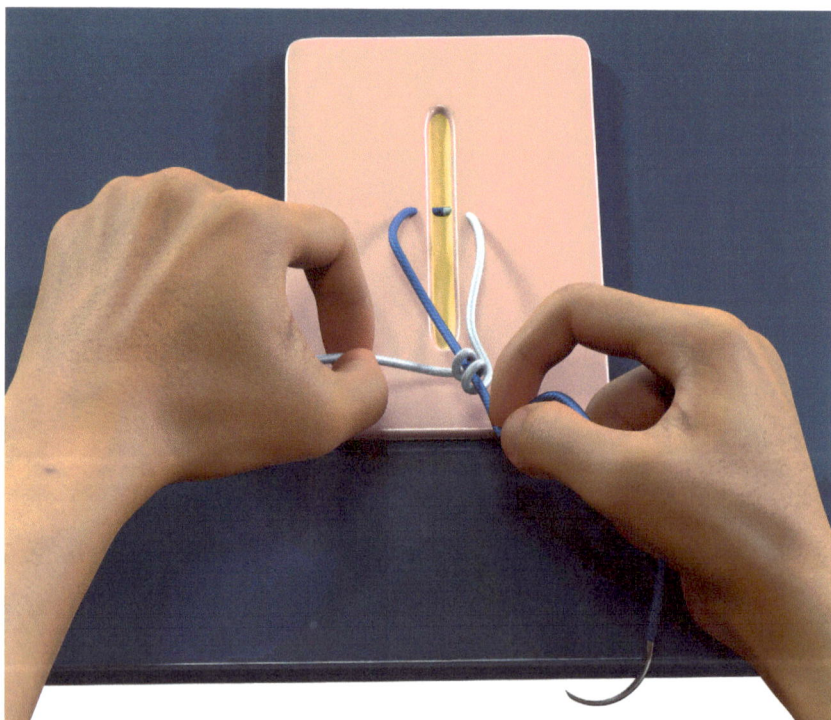

Step 7: Wrap the short end around the loop with your right hand.

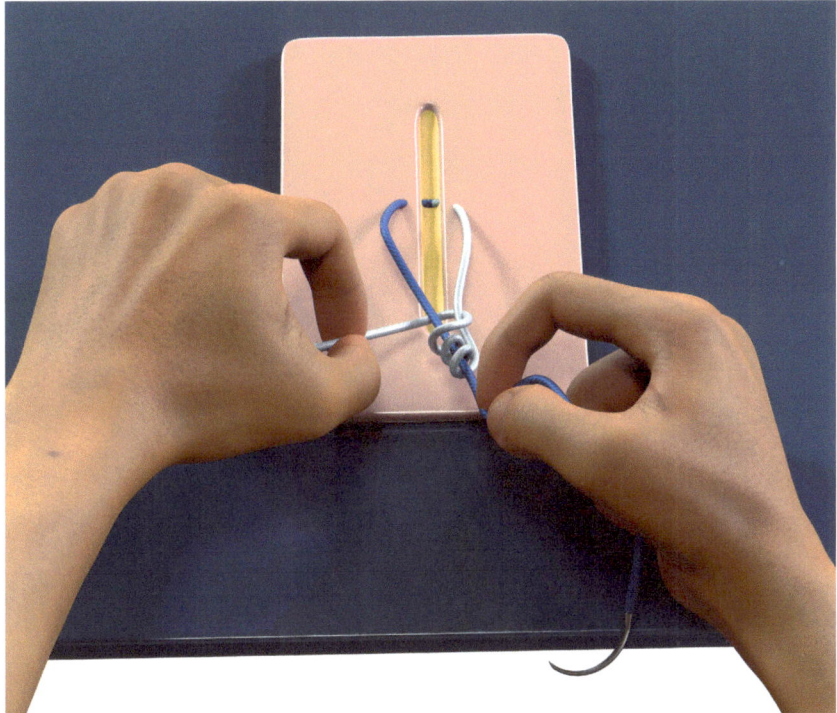

Step 8: Wrap the short end around the long end, away from the loop.

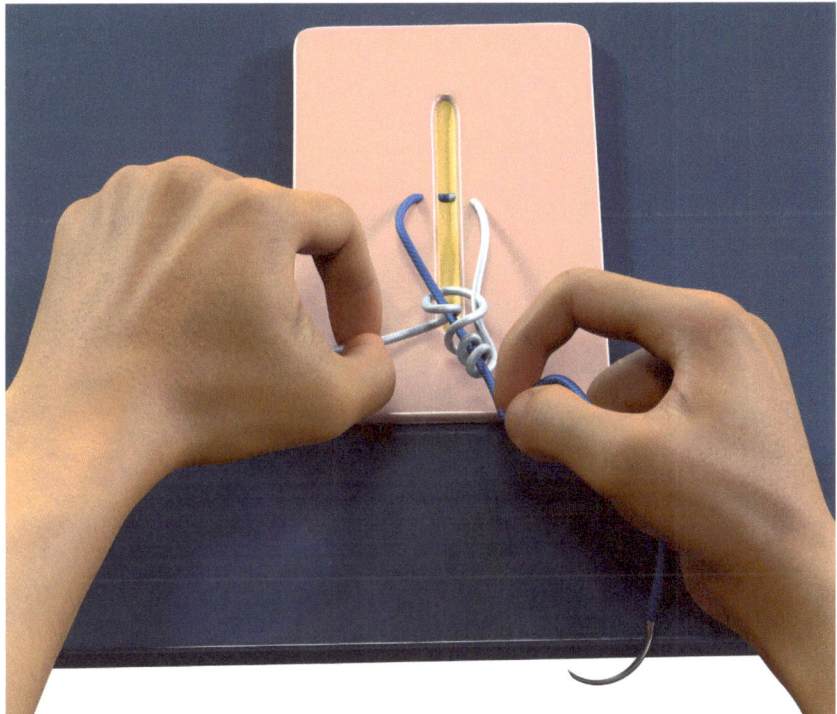

Step 9: Place the short end of the suture downward around the long end of the suture closer to your left hand.

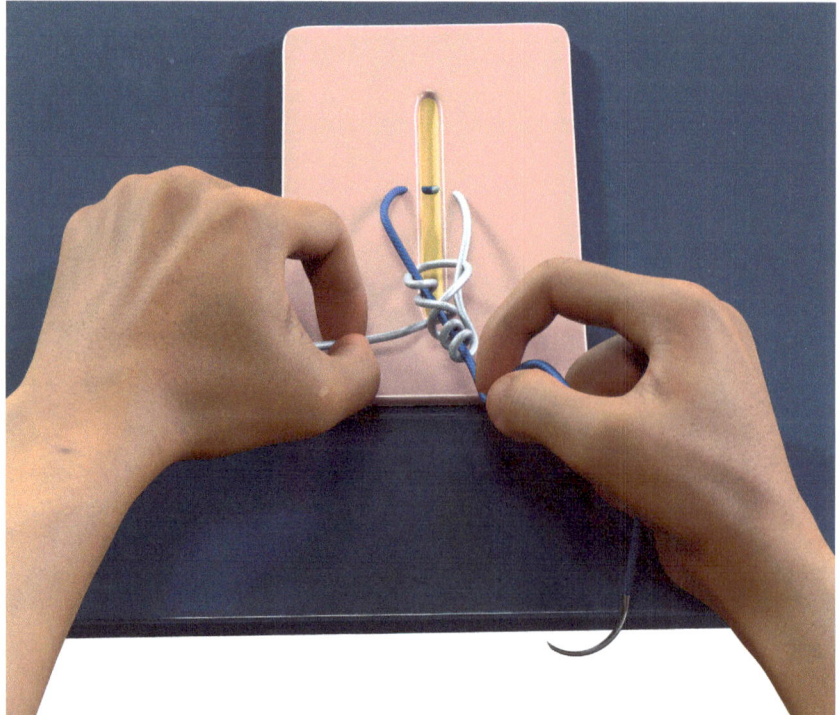

Mishra knots

Dr. R. K. Mishra at the World Laparoscopy Hospital in Gurgaon, India, developed two extracorporeal knots which are bulky but reported to be secure [70, 71]. Few publications have compared these knots with other extracorporeal knots for security and resistance to widening.

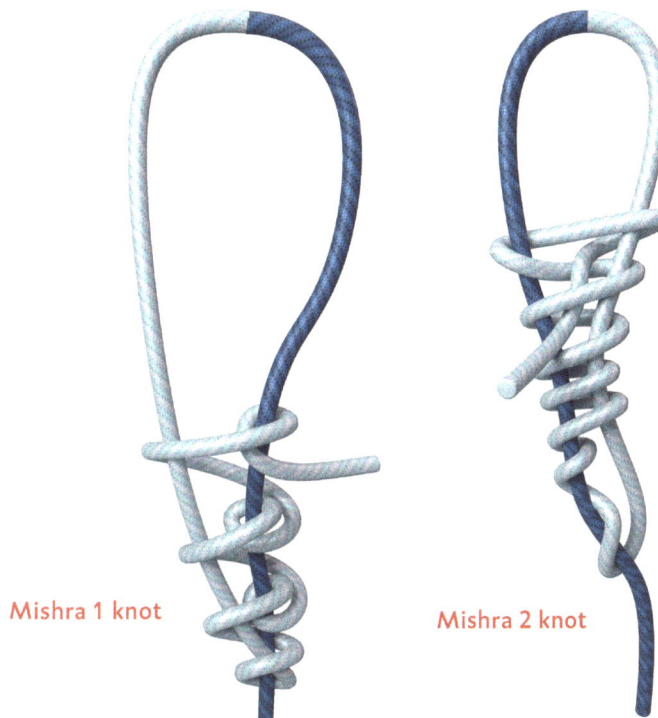

Mishra 1 knot   Mishra 2 knot

The Mishra knot 1 is formed by alternating half hitches around the post limb distally and wrapping around both portions of the loop for a total of three wraps and four half hitches. The Mishra knot 2 is formed similarly to the Melzer knot for steps 1 and 2, but instead of adding two half hitches, a Figure Eight knot is added at the end. The second knot appears more resistant to slipping than the original knot.

Knots commonly used in arthroscopy

In addition to extracorporeal knots previously discussed, nooses with partial locking ability frequently used in arthroscopy include the Duncan [11, 39, 40, 72], Tayside [39, 41], Pretzel [11, 67], Giant [11, 39, 67], and Weston [39, 40, 62] knots.

The Nice knot is particularly resistant to stretching. It has a double strand of suture around the tissue and is frequently used in orthopedic surgery as cerclage for humerotomy or femorotomy. The Nice knot uses a looped needle for suturing, generally with braided polyester [11].

Some orthopedic services have developed their own locking or friction knots (such as the Wiese and West Point knots, the latter being similar to the Arthroscopic Duncan Loop) [39]. Often these knots have had little scientific scrutiny in comparison with other arthroscopic knots [64, 73].

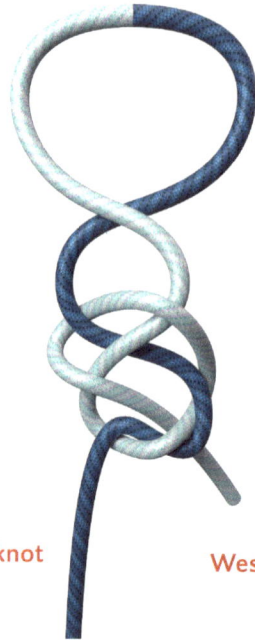

Wiese knot

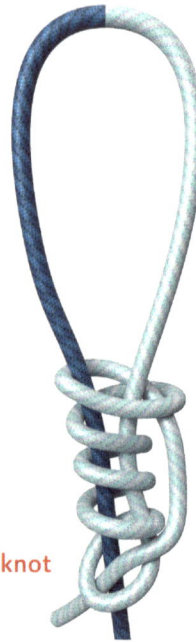

West Point knot

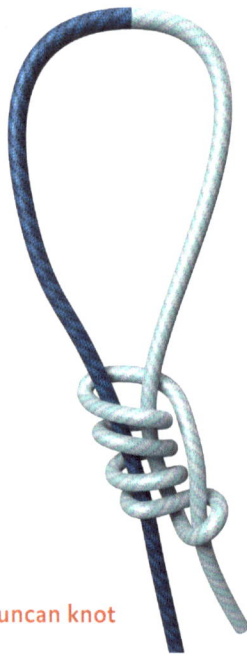

Duncan knot

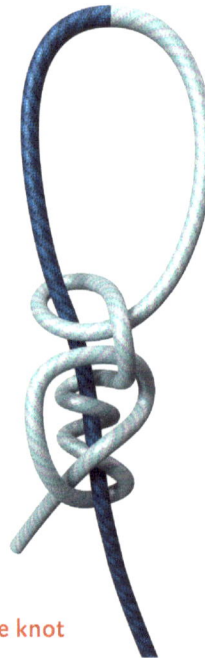

Tayside knot

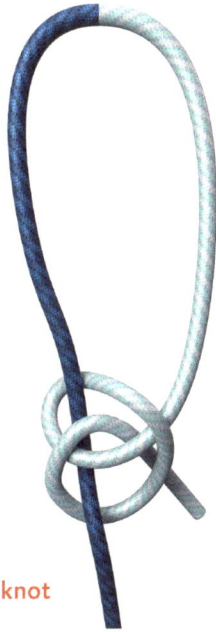

Pretzel knot

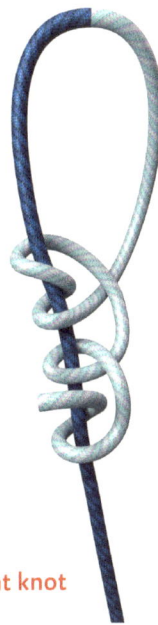

Giant knot

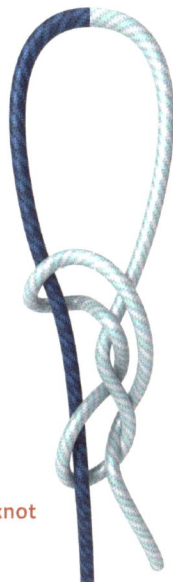

Weston knot

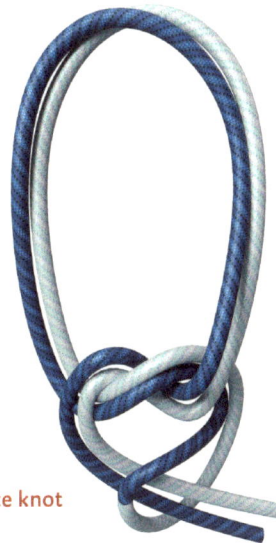

Nice knot

Comparison of knots

There is a moderate chance of slippage for extracorporeal and arthroscopic knots tied by both residents and experienced attendings, regardless of which knot is used, even when reversed half hitches on alternating posts are used to secure the knots [74]. The relative security of various knots depends on the type and size of the suture and how security is defined. Locking knots, for instance, have a high resistance to slippage, but the flipping of the knot during locking may result in it not being as tight as reversed half hitches on alternating posts.

Ratcheting knots

Shimi et al. [45] compared the security of the Tayside, Roeder, Melzer, Cross Square, and Blood knots using 0 and 2-0 silk, Polyamide, Dacron, PDS, and Polysorb sutures. In their study, knots were slipped and then tied flat, with tying tension standardized. Security was measured with a tensiometer to the point of slippage or breakage. The authors also measured strain (stretch/original length). They found that with Dacron and Lactomer, the Tayside, Melzer, and Roeder knots worked best. However, with PDS suture, the Melzer and Tayside, but not Roeder knots, were reliable. Silk and Polyamide were not secure with any of the knots tested. The force required to reverse the slipping of nooses was about twice for 0 compared with 2-0 suture. This study used a tapered cone to test force to slippage or breakage. The Tayside knot had an extra twist, but the Melzer lacked an additional half hitch at the end. The Tayside and Melzer were tied to 50 kg, while others were tied to 5 kg. The study postulated that arterial closure required 5 N force to be secure.

Flat knots versus nooses

Zimmer et al. [26] compared the Square, Granny, Surgeon's, and Square nooses using 5-0 monofilament and polyfilament Nylon suture. They tied knots to 80% holding power around a 38 mm cylinder with a 3 mm tail past the knots. Both slow and fast force stresses were applied, and videos were recorded of the knots to determine slippage or breakage. They found that the Square, Granny, and Surgeon's knots had the same security when tied down flat. All flat knots were significantly more secure than a noose.

Double wrapped knots versus Surgeon's knot

Taylor et al. [25] tested the Constrictor, Surgeon's, Modified Surgeon's, Strangle, and Modified Millers using 3-0 Proline, Polyglactin (Vicryl), Polydioxone (PDS), and Poliglecaprone (Monocryl) suture. They measured the force for a ligator to slip down a rod after knots were tied to 5, 10, or 15 N. They found that, although security was similar when using PDS suture for Constrictor, Strangle, and Miller knots, the Constrictor knot retained tension the best with PDS suture. Polyglactin kept tension the least.

Flat knots

Zhao et al. [1] tested the TSOL knot, three-throw Square, four-throw Square, one-throw Surgeon's, and two-throw Surgeon's knots using 3-0 braided polyblend (FiberWire), Polydioxanone (PDS), and Polyester (Ethibond) sutures. Knots were tied around a 30 mm rod to a load of 1 kg with 3 mm ends. The hydraulic force needed to cause slippage or breakage was measured. They found that the TSOL knot had a higher force to fail than the four Square knots for Fiberwire, PDS, and Ethibond. (P<0.05).

Nooses

Baumgarten et al. [39] tested the Double Twist knot, Tennessee Slider, Snyder's knot, Revo knot, SMC knot, Duncan knot, and various Roeder knots using Ethibond, Ticron, and PDS II suture. Since this paper summarized multiple studies, the only methodology reviewed was "load to clinical failure." They found that the Roeder knot was less secure than the Duncan or Square knot with Ticron. The Revo Knot was better than SMC or Duncan knots with Ethibond Number-2. They found no significant differences in failure using PDS sutures among various Roeder knots, the Revo knot, and the Square knot.

Comparison of orthopedic knots

P. Lacroix et al [66] compared knot tying with the Tennessee slider, Duncan loop, Revo knot, Nicky Knot, and SMC knot in a simulation lab among ten orthopedic residents. They measured both the ease of learning and reliability of the knots. The Revo knot was the easiest to learn but the Nicky knot had the highest reliability. The overall success rate for the knots was 80%. In another small study of 16 orthopedic residents, [75] the SMC, Weston, and Surgeon's knots were compared. The SMC knot was the most reliable in this comparison and the authors recommended that tying this knot should be incorporated into orthopedic training programs.

Ratcheting versus locking knots

Karahan et al. [67] tested the Pretzel, SMC, Giant, Dines, Nicky's knot, and Tennessee Slider using #2 Ethibond braided polyester suture. Failure was tested both with load to failure and cyclic loading. Each knot was loaded to 7 N around a 13.4 mm cylinder with 3-5 mm tags to knots. Cyclic loading used 7 and 30 N for 200 cycles. Knots loaded to failure at a strain rate of 1.25 mm/sec. The Pretzel knot had lower loop elongation compared with SMC and Dines knots. The Nicky and Tennessee Slider knots failed at low loads. The maximum loop elongation with cyclic loading was better with Giant and Dines knots than with the SMC or Pretzel knots. Load to failure was not significantly different among knots. The authors recommended backing up all knots with three reverse half hitches on alternating posts. The Pretzel and Dines knots had the least elongation with cyclical loading when additional half hitches were used.

Ratcheting knots with and without added half hitches

Lo et al. [40] tested the Duncan, Nicky's knot, Tennessee Slider, Roeder, SMC, and Weston knots with and without three half hitches on alternating posts, using #2 Ethibond and Fiberwire sutures. Knots were tied around a 30 mm post to a preload of 5 N. They measured force to failure, defined as 3 mm displacement or breakage, and found that the Weston Knot had the largest force to failure of nooses without reverse half hitches on alternating posts. The Roeder knot was second best for both suture materials. The Duncan, Roeder, Weston, and Tennessee Slider knots elongated more than 3 mm with the load. The Roeder knot had less suture loop enlargement than the SMC knot. The Revo knot was the most secure. These researchers found that adding three reverse half hitches on alternating posts improved the knot security of all sliding knots. However, the Roeder knot was tied very differently than is described in most studies.

Ligation of a blood vessel

Hazenfield et al. [30] tested the Miller, Constrictor, and Strangle knots using 2-o polyglyconate suture. Knots were tied to a force of 19.61 N for 10 seconds around a balloon dilation catheter. The dilation catheter was distended to measure the security of the knots. They found that all knots tested had excellent security and all were better than a Surgeon's knot for vascular pedicles. The Surgeon's and modified Miller's knots slipped at pressures below arterial pressure. The Constrictor had the best security at high pressures.

Roeder versus Gea knot

Moreno et al. [69] tested the Gea and Roeder knots using 1-o Polypropylene, Silk, Catgut, Polyglycolic acid, and Polyglactin 910 sutures, using a tensiometer to measure slippage or breakage. They found that the Gea knot had less slippage than the Roeder for Polyglactin 910 or Polypropylene sutures. They also reported that the Roeder knot was secure for suture diameters < 3 mm but not for greater diameters. In this study, there was no standardization of tying tension.

SMC versus Weston and Surgeon's knot

The University of Kentucky [75] compared the SMC with the Weston and Surgeon's knots, arthroscopically tied by orthopedic surgery residents at various levels in their training. They looked at how much force was required to cause knot failure and found that the SMC knot failed at significantly higher loads than the Surgeon's and Weston knots. The magnitude of force needed for knot failure did not differ between residents at different levels in their training or when compared with sports medicine fellows.

Chapter 9: Intracorporeal Laparoscopic Knots

Intracorporeal knots are best tied with braided suture using a Square noose technique, with additional flat throws for security. Intracorporeal suturing is a complex skill and best learned in a simulation lab. Proper port placement is crucial - creating a baseball diamond configuration with the camera on second base, the trocars on first and third base, and the knots and suturing at home base. Braided sutures are the best choice for intracorporeal knots. The sutures should be cut to 7 inches for interrupted knots and up to 10 inches for running sutures. Several techniques can be used: C loop outer or inner wraps, D loop, winding of suture around a laparoscopic needle holder [76], and intracorporeal one-handed. Ideally, the suture itself should be grasped to tie the knot. If the suture is too short, you can grasp the needle to perform the wraps, but this increases the risk of puncturing tissue with the tip of the needle.

C Loop: outer wrap intracorporeal

The C loop technique is the method preferred by 90% of laparoscopic surgeons, as it is easy to learn and faster than other methods [46, 77]. It is the method taught by SAGES and used in technical proficiency examinations for graduating general surgical residents.

Step 1: This is a reversed instrument tie, where you switch between the instruments held by your right and left hands to tie the knots. Begin by suturing through the tissue and then form a loop [41].

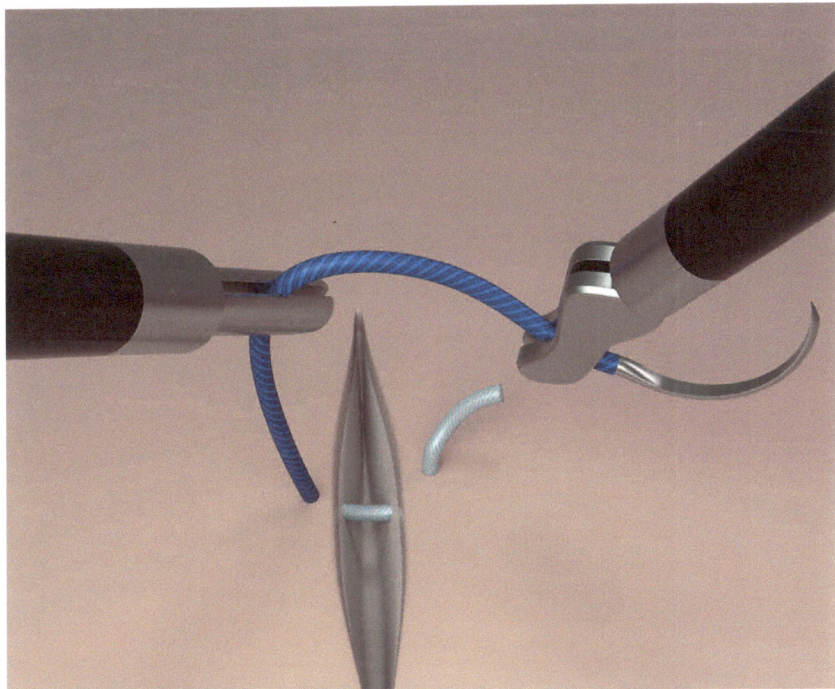

Step 2: With the needle holder in your right hand, wind the suture around the instrument in your left hand (once if Square knot, twice if Surgeon's), looping the suture counterclockwise (looking from the handle of the left-hand grasper towards its tip).

Make sure that the suture held with the instrument in your right hand is in front of the free end of the suture. Grasp the free end with the left grasper and pull it to the left to form a knot.

Step 3: With the instrument in your left hand, grasp the short end of the suture and pull it down flat.

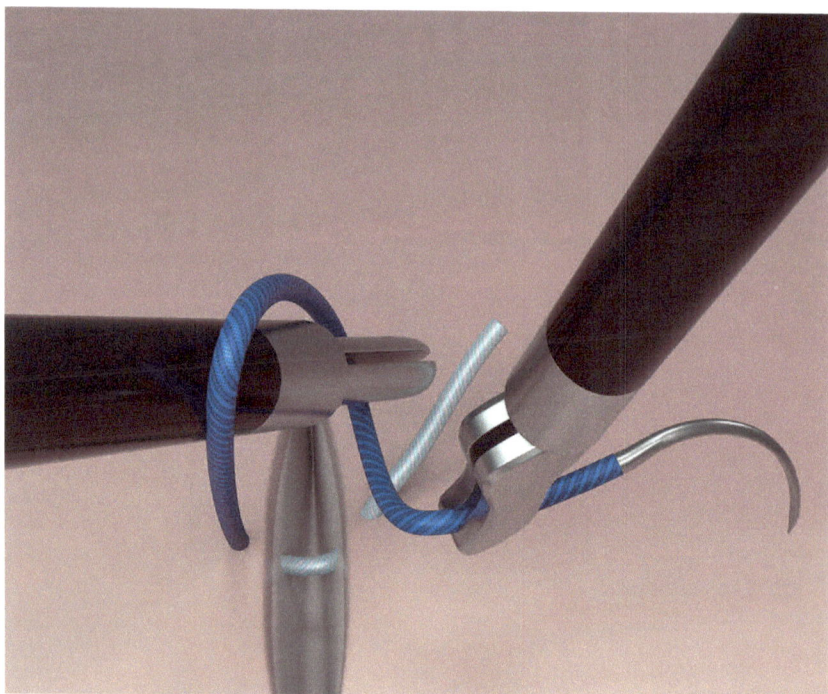

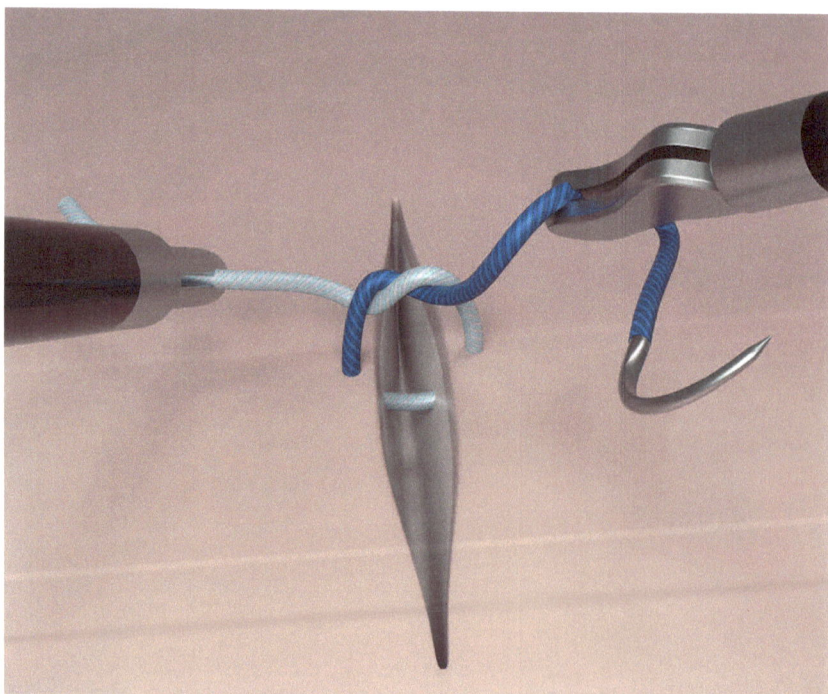

Step 4: Let go of the short end and grasp the long end of the suture with the instrument in your left hand. Make sure the suture forms a loop by pulling it with your needle holder.

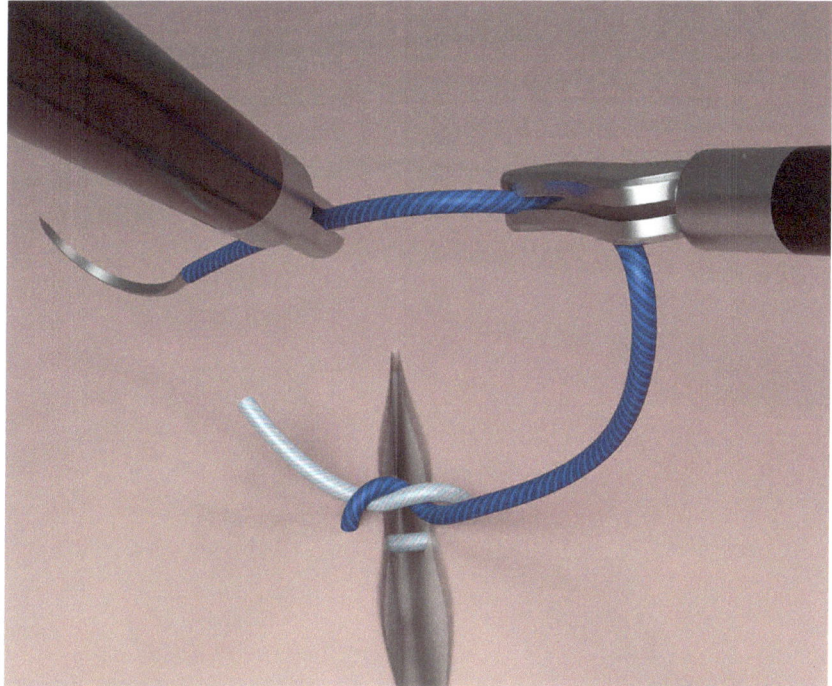

Step 5: Using the grasping instrument in your left hand, wrap the suture around the needle holder in your right hand.

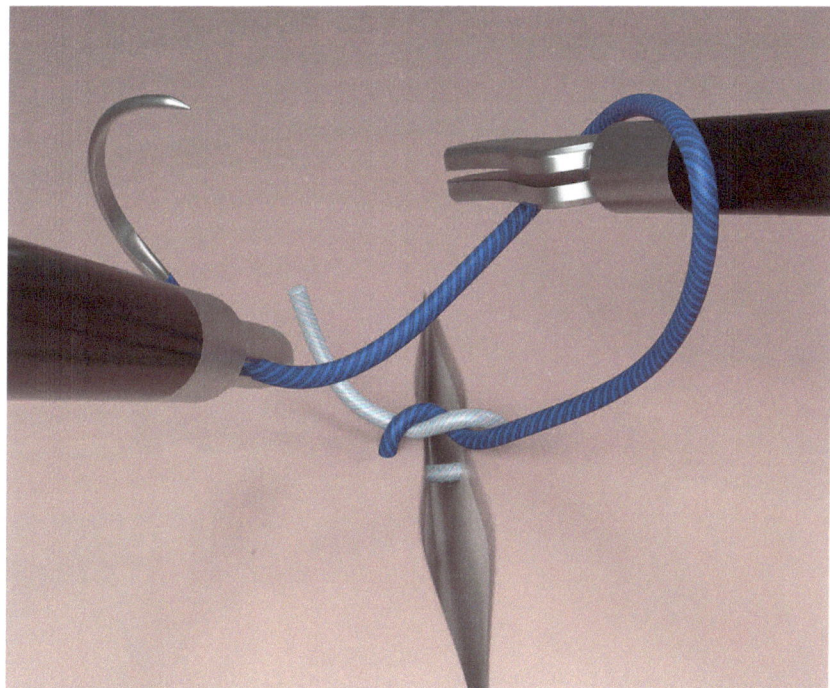

Step 6: Grasp the short end of the suture and pull it through.

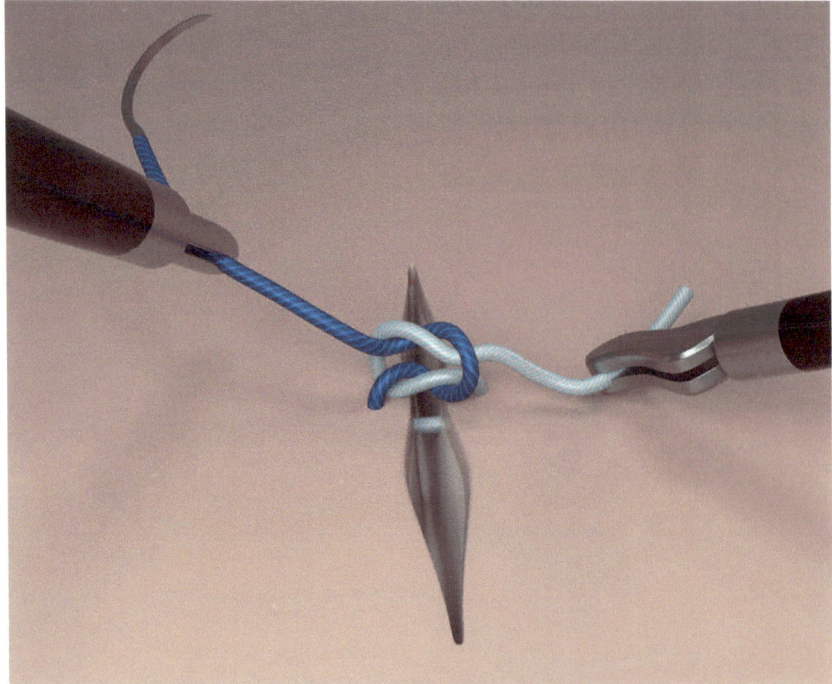

Step 7: Pull on the long end of the suture and the loop on the same side to change the Square knot to a noose.

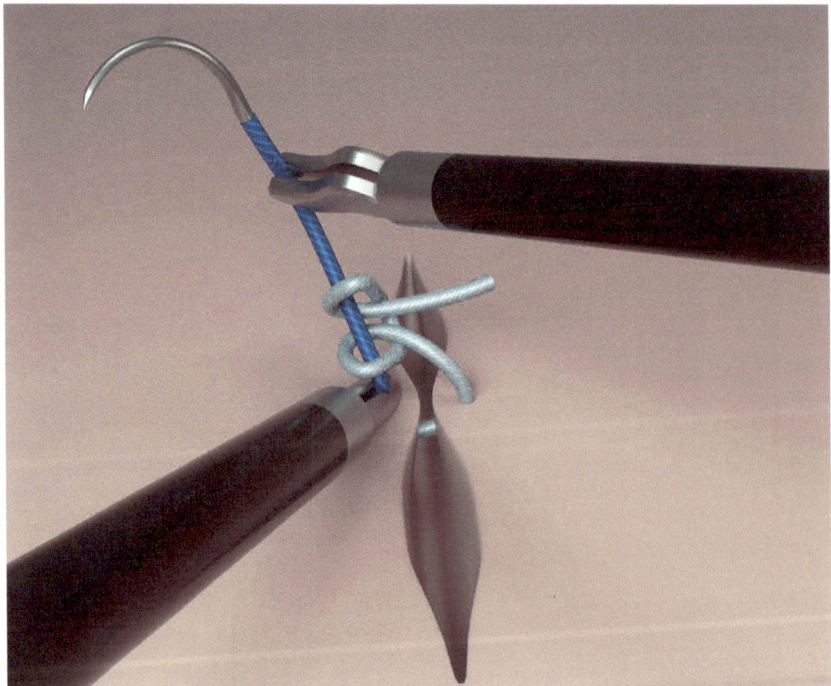

Step 8: Tighten the noose and then pull on the short end to lock it.

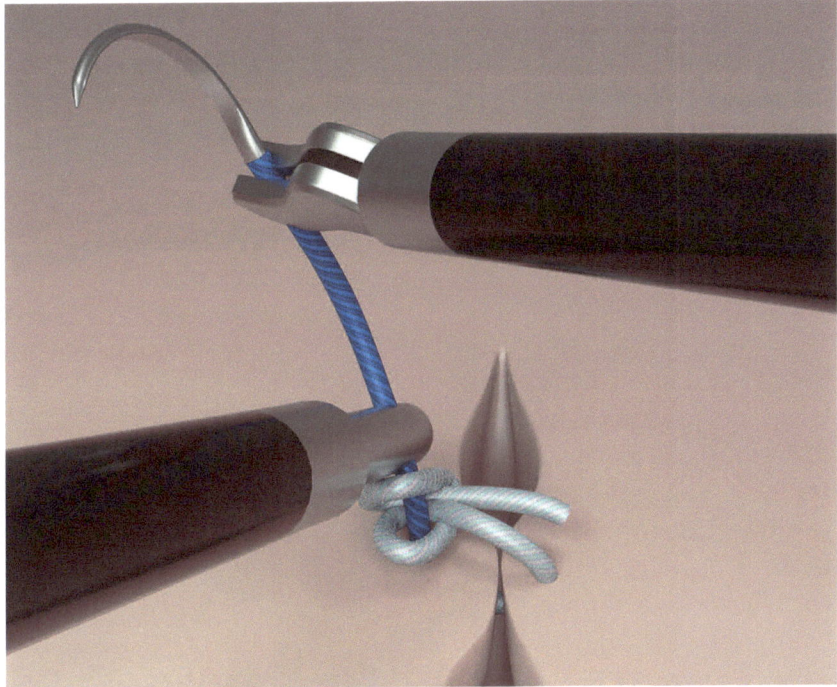

Step 9: Add additional Square knots as needed for security.

C Loop: inner wrap intracorporeal

The C loop inner wrap technique is closely related to the C loop outer wrap. It is a non-reversed instrument tie where you tie the knot alternating between using instruments held by your right and left hands [78, 79].

Step 1: Suture through the tissue and then form a loop. Wrap the suture clockwise (looking from the handle of the left-hand grasper towards its tip) around the instrument in your left hand (unlike the outer C loop technique, where the suture is wrapped counterclockwise).

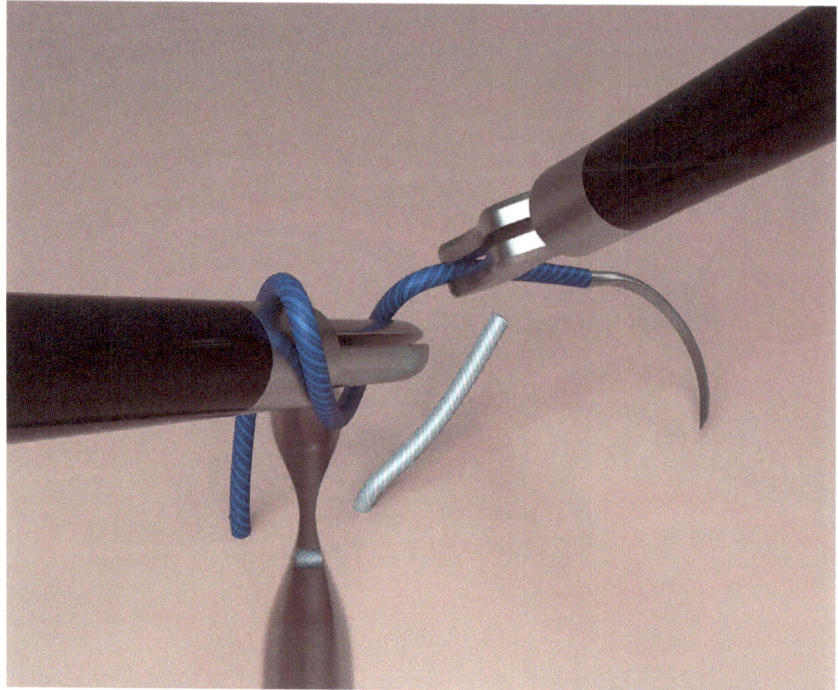

Step 2: Subsequent throws are similar to the outer wrap C loop technique, but the suture is wrapped around the instrument in the opposite direction.

D loop intracorporeal

The D loop intracorporeal method is a more complicated alternative to the C loop technique [80].

Step 1: The right-hand grasper holds the long end of the suture, and the left-hand grasper holds the suture 5 cm away. This technique requires a slightly longer suture, approximately 9-10 inches.

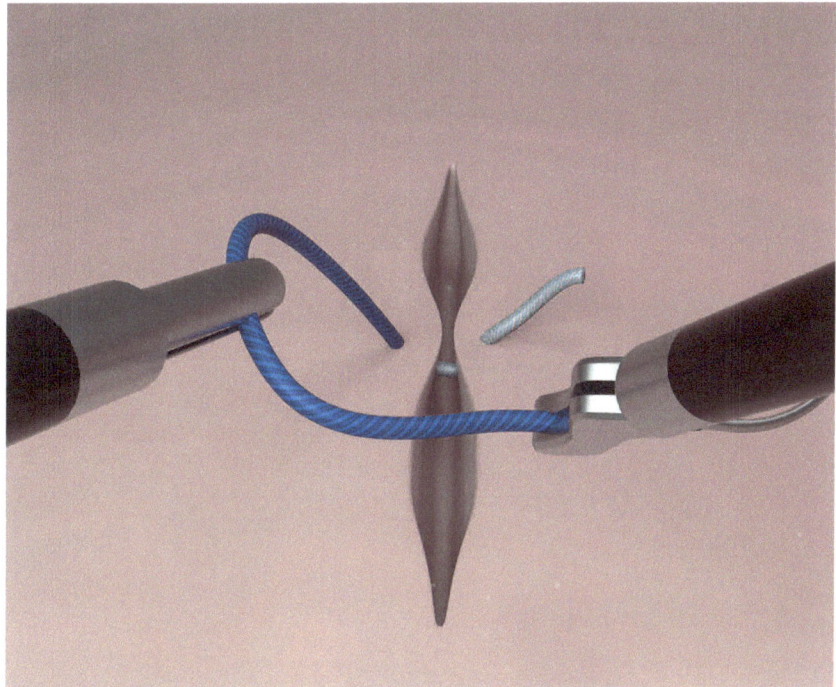

Step 2: Pull the suture down with the left-hand grasper. Push the long tail underneath with the right-hand grasper to form a "D" loop with the suture.

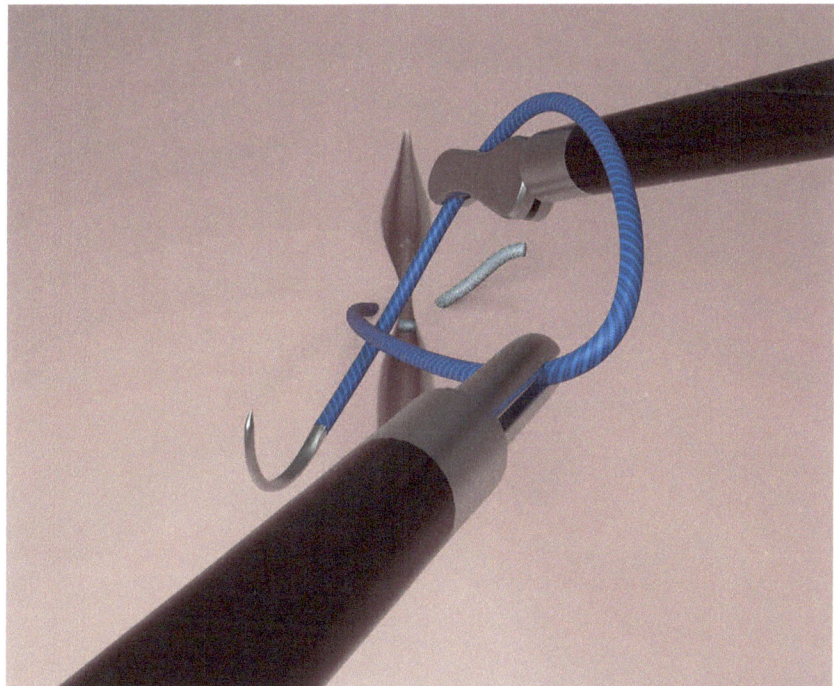

Step 3: Release the suture with the left grasper and grab the short end of the suture.

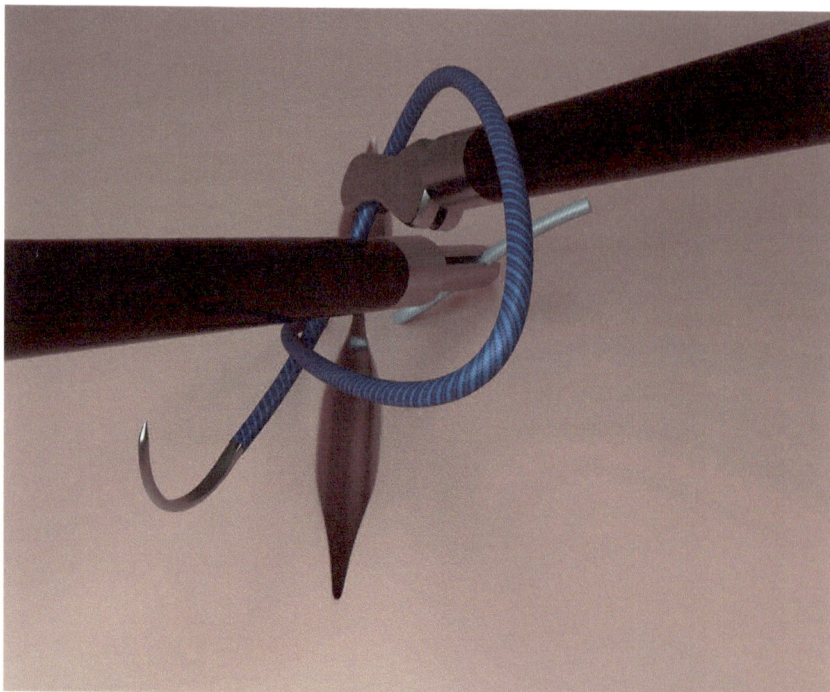

Step 4: Pull the suture through the loop and push the short end to make the knot lie down flat.

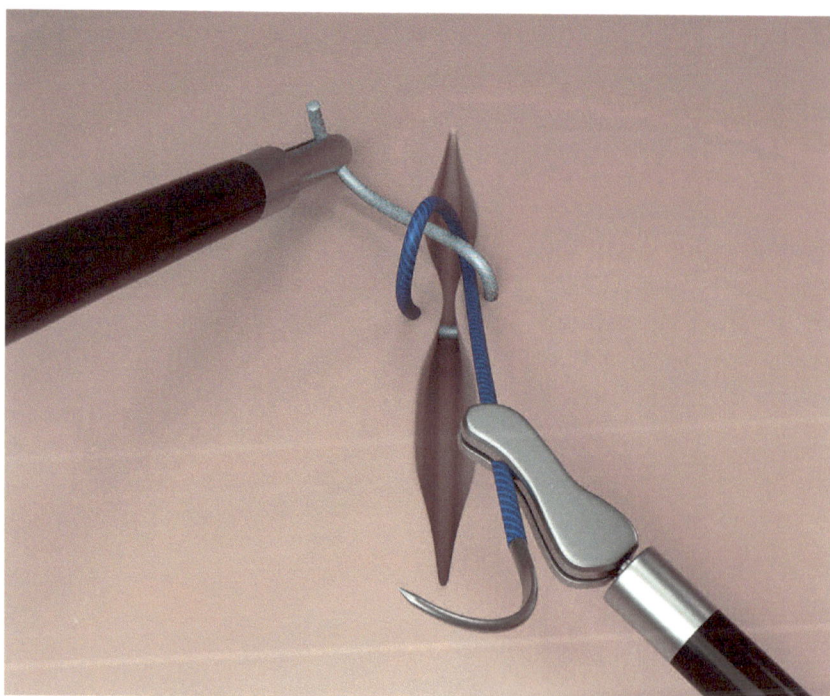

Step 5: Grab the long end with the two graspers.

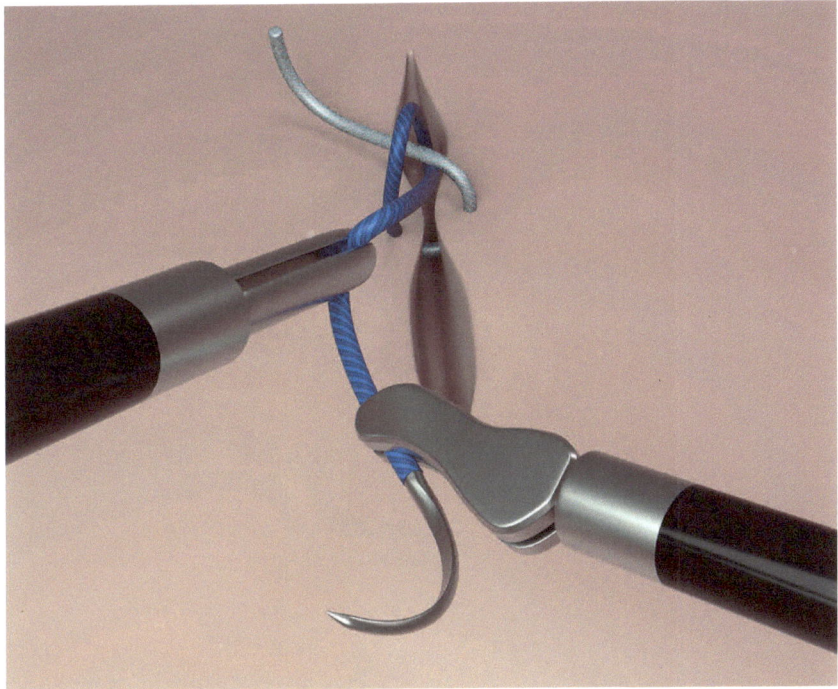

Step 6: Create a "reverse D" loop by pulling the loop to the left with the left grasper and the suture end to the right with the right grasper.

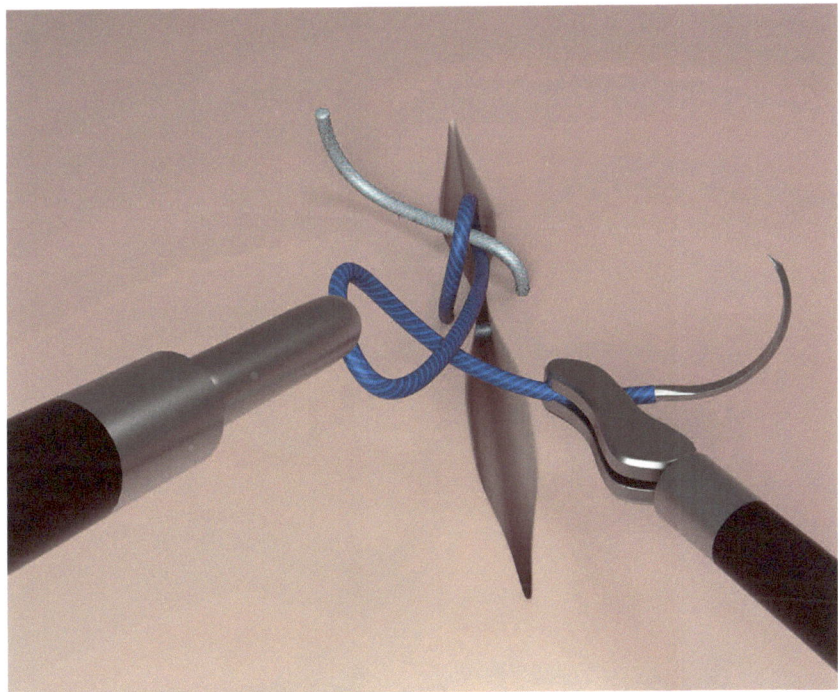

Step 7: Release the suture in the left grasper and use that instrument to grasp the short end of the suture.

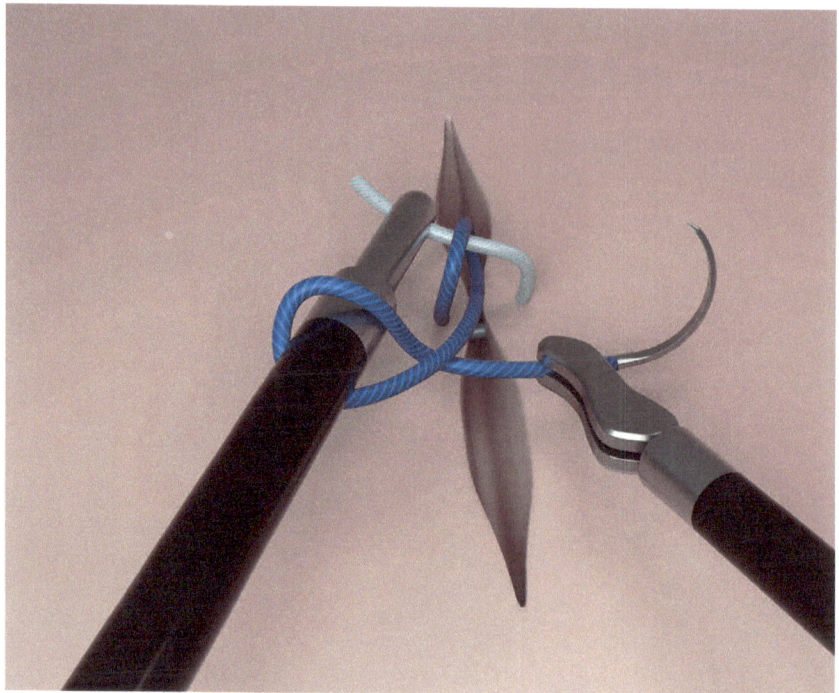

Step 8: Pull through to create the second knot.

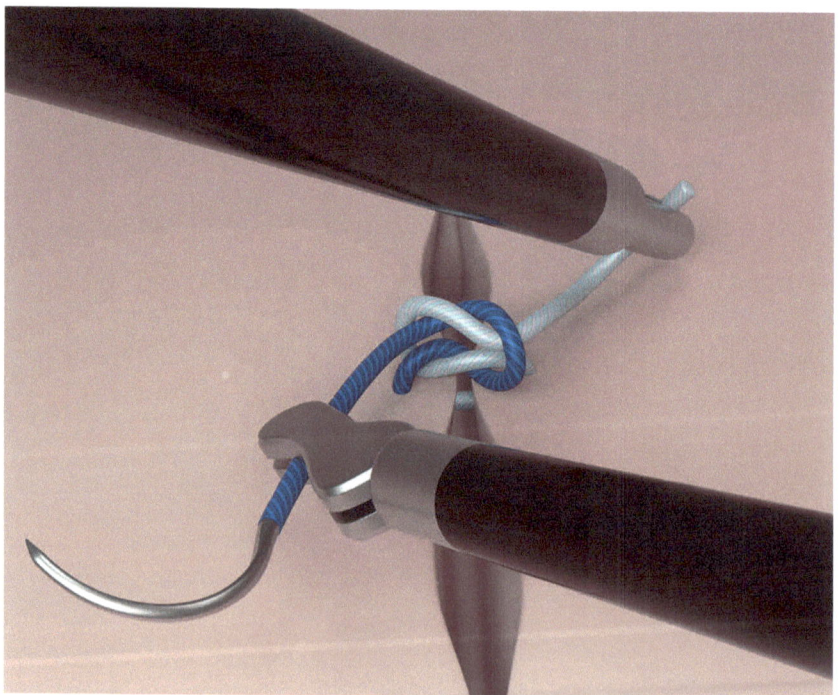

Winding intracorporeal

The winding technique is easy to learn for less experienced surgeons compared to the C loop technique and is functional in situations requiring very narrow angles of instrument manipulation [81,82]. A disadvantage of this technique is that the suture is grasped by the instrument, potentially weakening it. In tests using a laparoscopic simulator, the winding technique was slower than the one-handed intracorporeal method [76].

Step 1: This technique is best done with a right-angle clamp. Grasp the suture with the instrument in your left hand and spin the instrument counterclockwise until two loops of suture wrap around the instrument. Release the grasp on the suture loop and grab the suture's short end with the instrument in your left hand.

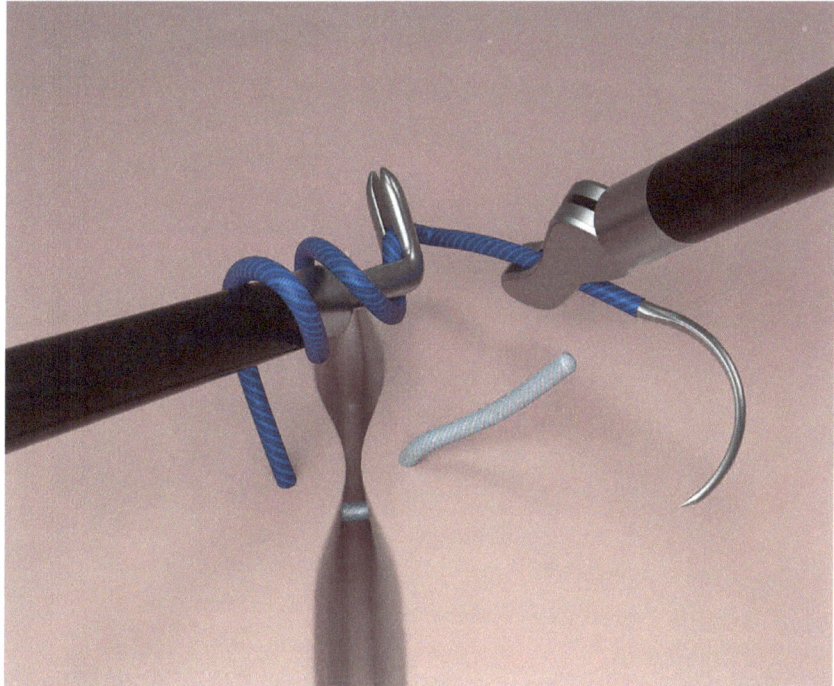

Step 2: For subsequent ties, spin the instrument, alternating clockwise and counterclockwise, wrapping one loop of suture around the instrument. Release and grab the short end of the suture and pull it in opposite directions for each throw.

One-hand intracorporeal

The one-hand intracorporeal technique can be used as an alternative to extracorporeal knot tying. It is tied like an open one-hand Square knot [76] and can be used as an alternative to an extracorporeal knot if there is tension on the long end of the suture.

Step 1: Grasp the short end of the suture.

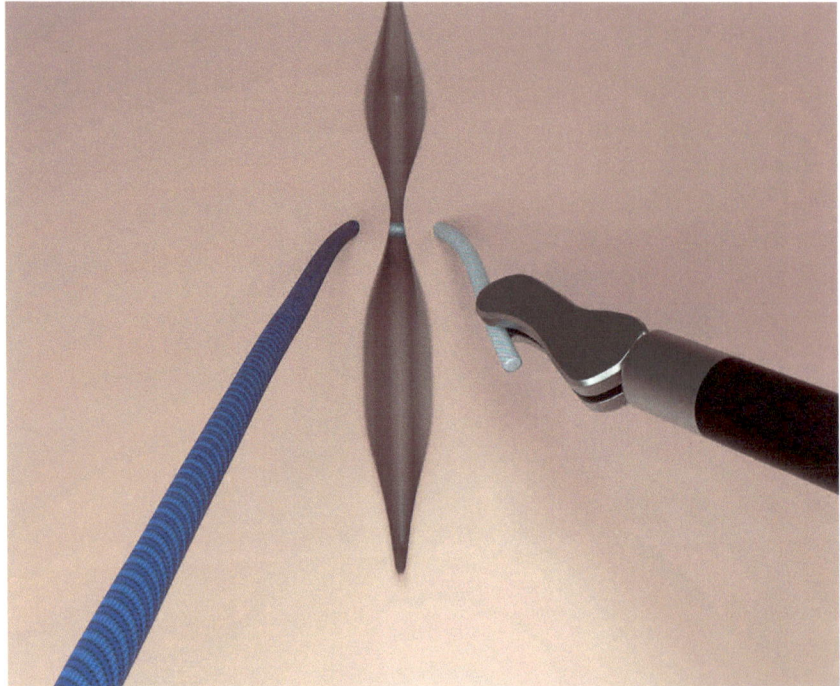

Step 2: Form a loop by pulling the short end across the top of the long end.

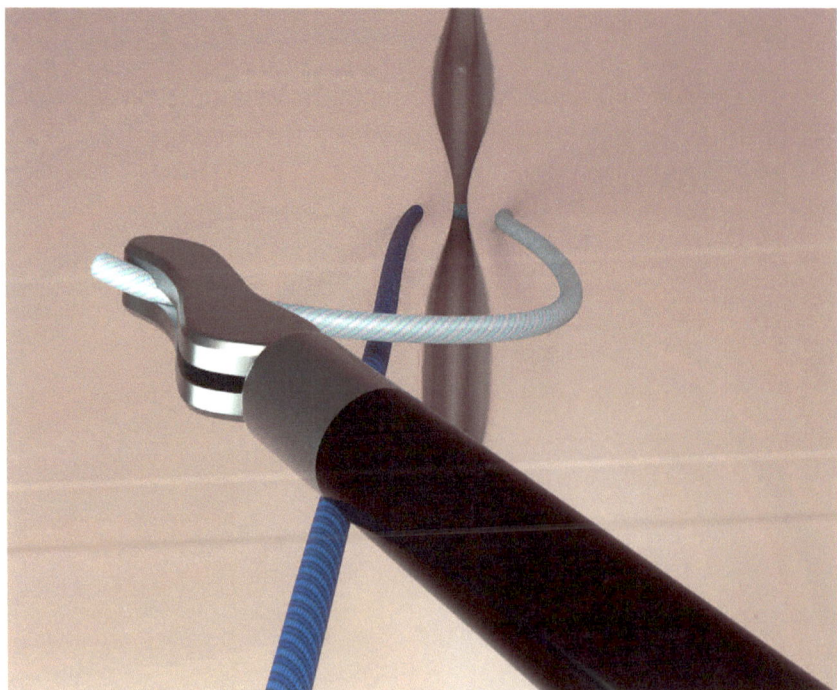

Step 3: Push the grasper through the loop.

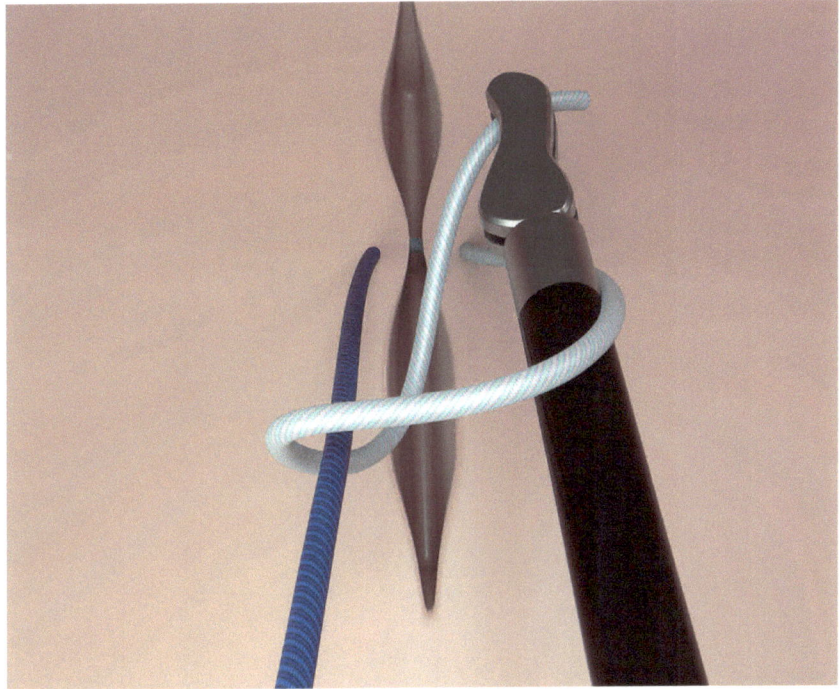

Step 4: Release the grasper and pull it back through the loop. Re-grasp the short end and pull it tight.

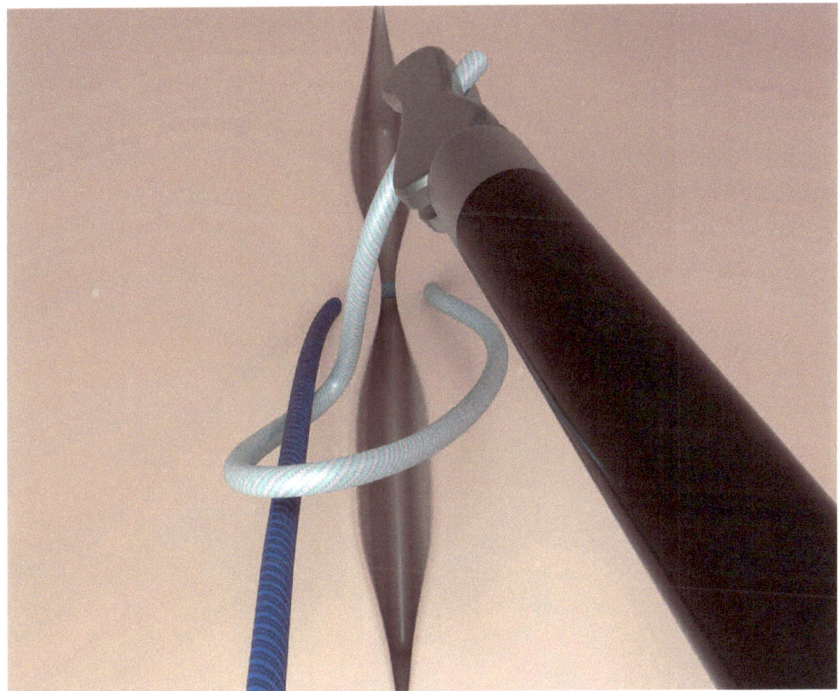

Step 5: Pull the short end of the suture behind the long end to create another loop.

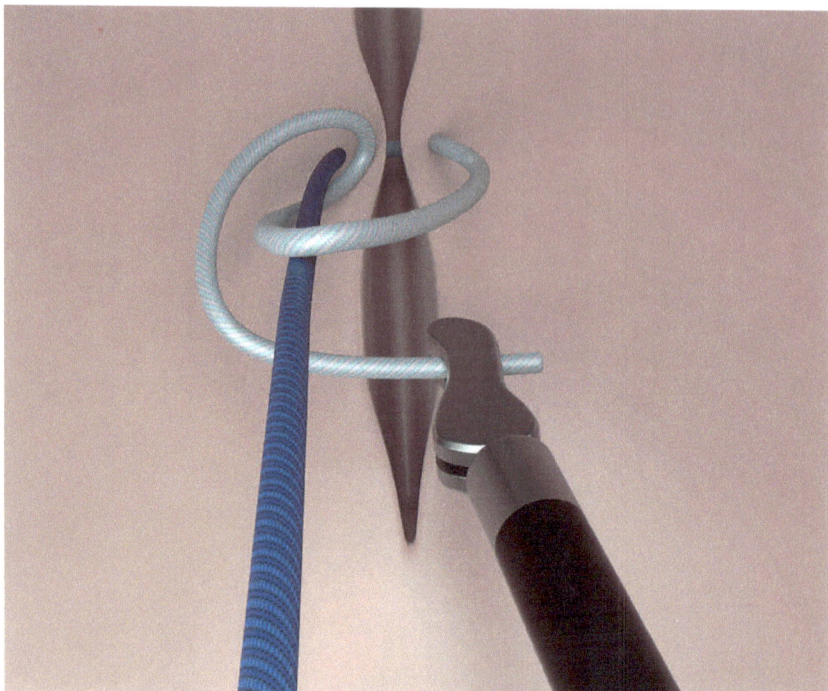

Step 6: Push the grasper through the loop, holding the short end.

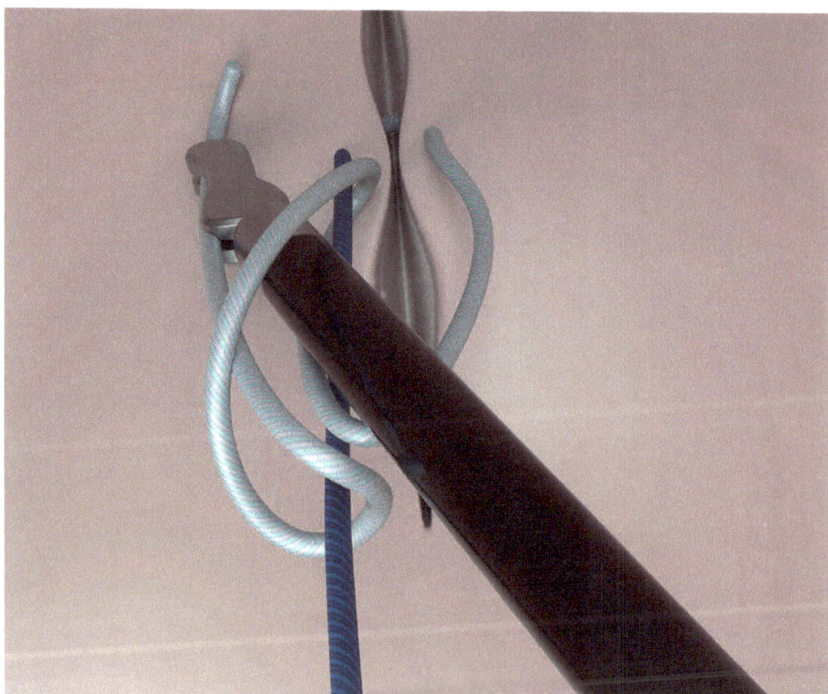

Step 7: Release the suture and pull the instrument back out of the loop. Re-grasp the short end of the suture and pull the knot down tight.

Bibliography

[1] Zhao C, Hsu C, Moriya T, et al. Beyond the Square knot: A Novel Knotting Technique for Surgical Use. *J Bone Joint Surg Am* 2013; 95:1020-7.

[2] Randall, P. The Craft of the Knot: From Fishing Knots to Bowlines and Bends. 2012, p 8.

[3] Hage, JJ. Heraklas on Knots: Sixteen Surgical Nooses and Knots from the First Century AD. *World J Surg* 2008; 32:648-655.

[4] http://emedicine.medscape.com/article/1127693-overview#a3

[5] Robinson JK, Hanke CW, Siegel DM, et al. Surgery of the Skin: Procedural Dermatology, third edition, Saunders, 2015.

[6] https://www.ethicon.com/na/products/wound-closure/absorbable-sutures/coated-vicryl-polyglactin-910-suture

[7] https://www.ethicon.com/na/products/wound-closure/absorbable-sutures/monocryl-poliglecaprone-25-suture

[8] https://www.ethicon.com/na/products/wound-closure/absorbable-sutures/PDS-ii-polydioxanone-suture

[9] https://www.medline.be/en/synthetic-absorbable-sutures-Maxon-Pointe-triangulaire-75-cm

[10] https://www.medline.be/en/synthetic-absorbable-sutures-Biosyn-2-0-24-mm-70-cm

[11] Akgun U, Karahan M, Randelli PS, Espregueira-Mendes J. Knots in Orthopedic Surgery: Open and Arthroscopic Techniques, Springer; 1st edition 2018.

[12] http://www.medscape.com/viewarticle/742992_7

[13] http://www.lightandmatter.com/article/knots.html

[14] Jawed MK, Dieleman P, Audoly B, Reis PM. Untangling the Mechanics and Topology in the Frictional Response of Long Overhand Elastic Knots. *Physical Review Letters* 2015; 115:118302.

[15] http://motherboard.vice.com/read/forget-dark-energy-physicists-have-finally-cracked-overhand-knots

[16] Friction and Friction Coefficients for various materials. https://www.engineeringtoolbox.com/friction-coefficients-d_778.html

[17] https://en.wikipedia.org/wiki/Capstan_equation

[18] http://www.jrre.org/att_frict.pdf

[19] https://www.scribd.com/document/354772602/IC-Sol-W03D1-4

[20] Gao X, Wang L, Hao X. An improved Capstan equation including power-law friction and bending rigidity for high performance yarn. *Mechanism and Machine Theory* 2015; 90:84-94.

[21] Warner C. Studies on the Behavior of Knots, in Turner JC, Van de Griend P, History and Science of Knots, 1996 World Scientific Publishing, pp. 181–203.

[22] Pieranski P, Kasa S, Dietler G, et al. Localization of breakage points in knotted strings. *New Journal of Physics* 2001; 3:10.1-10.13.

[23] Nigliazzo A, Arrangoiz R, Hutchison R, et al. Surgical Knot Strength in Continuous Wound Closures. *Surgical Science* 2011; 2:195-197.

[24] Aaning HI, Haas T, Jorgensen DR. Square Not a Running Knot. *J Am Coll Surg* 2007; 204: 422-425.

[25] Taylor H, Grogono AW, The constrictor knot is the best ligature. *Ann Royal College of Surgeons Engl* 2014; 96:101-105.

[26] Zimmer CA, Thacker JG, Powell DM, et al. Influence of Knot Configuration and Tying Technique on the Mechanical Performance of Sutures. *J of Emergency Med* 1991; 9:107-113.

[27] Turner JC, Van De Griend P. History and Science of Knots 1966; p5.

[28] Patil VP, Sandt JD, Kolle M, Dunkel J. Topological mechanics of knots and tangles. *Science* 2020; 367(6473):71-75.

[29] Ashley CW. The Ashley Book of Knots, 1944 Doubleday & Company; 1st edition 1993.

[30] Hazenfield KM, Smeak DD. In vitro holding security of six friction knots used as a first throw in the creation of a vascular ligation. *Journal of the American Veterinary Medical Association* 2014; 245(5):571-577.

[31] Leitch BJ, Kim NJ, Cann B, Lopez-Vilalobos N. Pedicle ligation in ovariohysterectomy: an in vitro study of ligation techniques. *Journal of Small Animal Practice* 2012; 53:592–598.

[32] Huber DJ, Egger EL, James SP. The Effect of Knotting Method on the Structural Properties of Large Diameter Nonabsorbable Monofilament Sutures. *Veterinary Surgery* 2004; 28:260-267.

[33] Muffy TM, Boyce J, Kieweg SL, Bonhom A. Tensile strength of a surgeon's or a Square knot. *J Surg Educ* 2014; 67(4):222-226.

[34] Trimbos JB. Security for Various Knots Commonly used in Surgical Practice. *Obstetrics & Gynecology* 1984; 64:274-280.

[35] Simonds, L. The Strongest Surgeon's Knot Strength Test [For Mono & Braid]. http://www.saltstrong.com/articles/surgeons-knot/

[36] Scott-Conner C. Chassin's Operative Strategy in General Surgery: An Expositive Atlas. 4th Edition 2013; page 37.

[37] https://www.climbing.com/skills/in-defense-of-the-european-death-knot/

[38] Wu V, Yeung C, Sykes EA, and Zevin B. Comparison of knot-tying proficiency and knot characteristics for square and reversing half hitch alternating-post surgical knots in a simulated deep body cavity among novice medical students. *Can J Surg* 2018; 61(6):385-391.

[39] Baumgarten KM, Wright RW. Arthroscopic Knot Tying: An Instruction Manual. 2005.

[40] Lo K, Burkart SS, Chan CC, Athanasiou K. Arthroscopic Knots: Determining the Optimal Balance of Loop Security and Knot Security. *J Arthroscopic and Related Surgery* 2004; 20(5):489-502.

[41] Akindele RA, Fasanu AO, Chandra S, Komolafe JO, Michra RK. Comparing Extracorporeal knots in Laparoscopy using Knot and Loop Securities. *World J Lap Surg* 2014; 7(1):28-32.

[42] Ilahi OA, Younas SA, Alexander J, Noble PC. Cyclic testing of arthroscopic knot security. *Arthroscopy* 2004; 20(1):62-8.

[43] Laitai GL, Snyder SJ, Applegate GR, et al. Shoulder Arthroscopy and MRI Techniques. Springer 2003; ISBN 3-540-43112-8.

[44] Gandini M, Guisto G, Comino F, Pagliara E. Parallel alternating sliding knots are effective for ligation of mesenteric arteries during resection and anastomosis of the equine jejunum. *BMC Vet Res* 2014; 10(1):s10.

[45] Shimi SM, Lirici M, Velpen GV, Chschieri A. Comparative study of the holding strength of slipknots using absorbable and nonabsorbable ligature materials. *Surg Endosc* 1994; 8:1285-1291.

[46] Soper NJ, Scott-Conner CE. The SAGES Manual, Volume 1: Basic Laparoscopy and Endoscopy, 3rd Edition. Springer Publishing 2012.

[47] https://www.theguardian.com/artanddesign/gallery/2019/dec/10/scientific-phenomena-photographs-of-the-year-in-pictures-royal-society-publishing#img-15

[48] Behm T, Unger JB, Mekherjee D. Flat Square knots: are 3 throws enough? *Am J Obstetrics and Gynecology* 2007; 197(2):172e1-172e3.

[49] Tidwell JE, Vincent LK, Samora JB. Knot Security: How Many Throws Does It Really Take? *Orthopedics* 2012; 35(4):e542-537.

[50] Drake DB, Rodeheaver PF, Edlich RF, Rodeheaver GT. Experimental studies in swine for measurement of suture extrusion. *J Long Term Eff Med Implants* 2004;14(3):251-9.

[51] Kim E, Chern H, Huang E, Palmer B. How to teach knot tying: teaching with the kinesthetic approach. University of California San Francisco, MedEdPORTAL publications 2013; 9:9328 (https://www.mededportal.org/publication/9328)

[52] Drabble E, Spanopoulou S, Sioka E, et al. How to tie dangerous surgical knots easily. Can we avoid this? *British Medical Journal Surg Interv Health Technologies* 2021; 3:e000091:1-10.

[53] https://www.animatedknots.com/constrictorretrieve/index.php

[54] Regier PJ, Smeak DD, Coleman K, McGilvray KC. Comparison of volume, security, and biomechanical strength of square and Aberdeen termination knots tied with 4–0 polyglyconate and used for termination of intradermal closures in canine cadavers. *Journal of the American Veterinary Medical Association* 2015; 247(3):260-266.

[55] Stott PM, Ripley LG, Lavelle MA. The Ultimate Aberdeen Knot. *Annals of The Royal College of Surgeons of England.* 2007; 89(7):713-717.

[56] Miyazaki D, Ebihara Y, Satoshi H. A New Technique for Making the Aberdeen Knot in Laparoscopic Surgery. *J Laparoendoscopic & Advanced Surg Tech* 2015; 25:499-502.

[57] https://www.youtube.com/watch?v=ieOo6_xt5ec

[58] https://www.flsprogram.org/wp-content/uploads/2014/03/Revised-Manual-Skills-Guidelines-February-2014.pdf

[59] Xu AA, Jian FZ, Su Y. Towards a better knot: Using mechanics methods to evaluate three knot-tying techniques in laparo-endoscopic single-site surgery. *J Minim Access Surg* 2015; 11(4):241-245.

[60] http://www.google.com/patents/EP0477020A1?cl=en

[61] Kim SH, Yoo JC, Wang JH, et al. Arthroscopic sliding knot: how many additional half-hitches are really needed? *Arthroscopy* 2005; 21(4):405-11.

[62] Hage JJ, Van der Steen LP. Locking, Jamming, and Ratchet Mechanisms of Sliding Surgical Knots Topologically Revisited. *World Journal of Surgery* 2009; 33(4):751–757.

[63] Hanypsiak BT, et al. Knot Strength Varies Widely Among Expert Arthroscopists. *Am J Sports Med* 2014; 2(8):1978-84.

[64] Parada SA, Shaw KA, Eichinger JK, et al. The Wiese Knot: A Sliding-Locking Arthroscopic Knot. *Arthroscopy Techniques* 2017; 6(1): e21-e24.

[65] Baums MH, Sachs C, Kostuj T, et al. Mechanical testing of different knot types using high-performance suture material. *Knee Surgery, Sports Traumatology, Arthroscopy* 2015; 23(5):1351-1358.

[66] Lacroix PM, Commeil P, Chauveaux D, Fabre T. Learning and optimizing arthroscopic knot-tying by surgical residents using procedural simulation. Orthop Traumatol Surg Res. 2021 12; 107(8): 102944.

[67] Karahan M, Akgun U, Turkoglu A, Nuran R, et al. Pretzel knot compared with standard suture knots. *Knee Surg Sports Traumatol Arthrosc* 2012; 20(11):2302-2306.

[68] Pereira-Graterol FA, Moreno-Portillo M. A New Technique for Tying the Gea Extracorporeal Endoscopic Knot for Endoscopic Surgery. *Journal of Laparoendoscopic & Advanced Surgical Techniques* 2004; 14(6):403-406.

[69] Moreno M, Magos FJ, Arcovedo R, et al. Comparison of the performance of the Gea Extracorporeal knot with the Roeder Extracorporeal knot and the Classical Knot. *Surg Endosc* 2004; 18:157-160.

[70] Mishra RK, Koruth S, Reshme N. Role of Mishra's Knots in Various Surgeries in Laparoscopy. *World J Lap Surg* 2016; 9(3):114-117.

[71] https://www.youtube.com/watch?v-JBV1k_fWpd8

[72] Alberta FG, Mazzoca AD, Cole BG, Roreo AA. Arthroscopic knot tying. Chapter 4, Textbook of Arthroscopy, WB Saunders, Elsevier Health Science Company 2003.

[73] Wolfe JA, Pickett AM, Blarcum GV, et al. The West Point Knot: A Sliding-Locking Arthroscopic Knot. *Arthroscopy Techniques* 2018; 7(7):e685-e689.

[74] Pedowitz RA, Nicandri GT, Angelo RL, et al. Objective Assessment of Knot-Tying Proficiency with the Fundamentals of Arthroscopic Surgery Training Program Workstation and Knot Tester. *Arthroscopy: The Journal of Arthroscopic and Related Surgery* 2015; 6(21):1-8.

[75] Cronin KJ, Cox JL, Hoggard TM, et al. The effect of residency training on arthroscopic knot tying and knot stability: which knot is best tied by Orthopaedic surgery residents? *Journal of Experimental Orthopaedics* 2018; 5(19):1-6.

[76] Romoni AP, Braasch M, Botnaru A, et al. Evaluation of Efficacy of Four Laparoscopic Needle Drivers. *J of the Society of Laparoendoscopic Surgeons* 2008; 2:77-80.

[77] Pennings JL, Kenyon T, Swanstrom L. The knit stitch: An improved method of laparoscopic knot tying. *Surg Endosc* 1995; 9:537-540.

[78] Cuschieri A, Szabo Z. Tissue Approximation in Endoscopic Surgery. Isis Medical Media, Oxford 1995.

[79] Nutan J. Laparoscopic Suturing. McGraw Hill Medical 2007; p 41.

[80] http://www.sages.org/wp-content/uploads/posters/2011/33197.jpg, https://www.youtube.com/watch?v=D-9K_VMjveM

[81] Thiyagarajan M, Ravindrakumar C. A Comparative Study in Learning Curves of Two Different Intra-corporeal Knot Tying Techniques. *Minimally Invasive Surgery* 2016: http://dx.doi.org/10.1155/2016/3059434

[82] Gopsidas, RR, Reul RM. Intra-corporeal Knot-Tying for the Thoracoscopic Surgeon: A Novel and Simplified Technique. *Texas Heart Institute Journal* 2010; 37(4):435-438.

Index

www.ingramcontent.com/pod-product-compliance
Lightning Source LLC
Chambersburg PA
CBHW041549260326

41914CB00016B/1593